I0022173

I HAVE MY
CAKE
AND EAT IT TOO

How Changing Your Thinking Can Help Win Your Health and Freedom

PEGGY FORNEY

The information in this book is provided to assist the reader in making informed choices about diet, exercise, and other life decisions. This book is not intended as a substitute for medical advice. Before starting any diet or physical activity, you should consult your personal physician. The author shall not be liable or responsible for any loss or damage allegedly arising from any information or suggestion in this book.

Copyright ©2012 Peggy June Forney
All rights reserved. Published in the United States by Forney Enterprises, Inc., Leadville, Colorado.

ISBN-13: 978-0-9857621-0-0
LCCN: 2012949383

Cover design by Brian Zimmerman at Cre843.

.

For Megan and Ashley

So that you and your families can have better lives

TABLE OF CONTENTS

ABOUT THE AUTHOR

You do not sell a fundamental change on the merits of the fundamental change.–Peggy June Forney

Peggy Forney spent twenty-three years working as marketing professional at Mountain Bell, AT&T, *U S WEST*, and Qwest. She has a bachelor's degree in Merchandising/Marketing and a Masters Degree in Technology Management. Her passion is enabling fundamental change.

In 1986, she cut her teeth on voice messaging when customers still hated talking to answering machines and clerks wrote pink message slips by hand. At *U S WEST*, Peggy alone saw the enormous market potential of voice messaging and she became a "Don Quixote" of sorts as she tried to get her executives to see her vision.

Stan Bader, Peggy's subsidiary president, was supportive which helped enable her to convince the board of directors to fund two trial Octel Communications voice messaging systems. Stan also defended Peggy's decision to purchase Octel equipment over VMX, the market leader at the time, to Jack MacAllister, the CEO of *U S WEST*. VMX had appealed her decision to the CEO of *U S WEST*.

Because voice messaging is a business product and generally rebranded, many consumers are unaware that Octel set the industry standard back in the 1980s and still sets the standard today. *U S WEST* was the first regional bell operating company to purchase Octel equipment. At the time Peggy made her decision, Octel was a small venture capital based company with approximately 150 employees. Octel purchased VMX for approximately $200 million in 1994. In 1997, Lucent Technologies acquired Octel for $2.1 billion. This dramatic growth of the voice messaging market is typical of fundamental change.

"Peggy's vision and tenacity was instrumental in the early adoption of voice mail at U S WEST which led to Octel's rapid growth." — Robert (Bob) Cohn, Co-founder of Octel Communications

In 1997, Peggy saw the enormous potential for DSL and she became the third person on the DSL marketing team. *U S WEST* was the first regional bell operating company to market DSL. As with all fundamental change, every early DSL sale was cause for celebration. The marketing message Peggy crafted for the techno-weenies was different than the one she crafted for the grandmas and grandpas. The experience that Peggy had gained from the early days of voice messaging came back into play again. As with voice messaging, DSL eventually reached critical mass, or Malcolm Gladwell's "Tipping Point," and DSL sales exploded. Today there are relatively few consumers who do not subscribe to some form of high speed internet.

In early 2004, Peggy came across a disturbing CDC (Centers for Disease Control) statistic and then took a long sobering look in the mirror and at her medical lab reports. What she saw in the mirror and on the lab reports confirmed the terrifying CDC statistic and the diagnosis from her doctor. It was undeniable that she was extremely obese, was insulin resistant, which meant she was one step away from becoming a type 2 diabetic, and that she would eventually develop heart disease. She would die young and there would be lots of pain and suffering before she died.

Peggy got fed up. It was time for a fundamental change. Peggy took two decades of experience enabling fundamental change and used it to figure out how to win her heath and freedom. *I Have My Cake and Eat It Too* is the result of what Peggy learned during her ninety pound weight loss journey and twenty-three years as a marketing professional.

"Peggy's inspirational weight loss and success at halting the progression of diabetes and heart disease makes me wish I had more patients like her." — Eric H. Leder, MD

INTRODUCTION

Every man is the creature of the age in which he lives; very few are able to raise themselves above the ideas of the time. —Voltaire (1694–1778)

The information in this book represents a li'l old (formerly) fat lady's attempt to help a few Americans raise themselves above the ideas of the time. Everything in this book comes from this perspective. A term you will see throughout this book is "turn the kaleidoscope." When you turn the kaleidoscope, it will help you raise yourself above the ideas of the time. When you turn the kaleidoscope, you are able to see what *can* be rather than what *is*.

While some of the conclusions are subjective, the underlying data sources are pristine. You are encouraged to read the scientific and government documents that were used to construct the logic and concepts that are presented. Many well-known nutrition expert book authors are also referenced. They represent the best of the best in medicine and science. All of the books can be obtained on Amazon.com. While reading the source documents and books constitutes an additional time and financial investment, the cost is tiny compared to the value you will receive.

The information in this book is divided into four parts. Part I explains what's wrong and some dietary fixes. Part II focuses on additional things that can increase our chances of regaining our health and personal freedom. Part III provides foods, recipes, and pearls of wisdom from the nutritional experts. And part IV offers some li'l old fat lady marketing strategies to help Americans get out of this terrible obesity and disease predicament.

Please read the pages of this book in order from the beginning to the end. Like building a house, the foundation must be completed before the roof is built. Without the foundation, there is no reference point for the roof, and the same is true for this book.

It is human nature to become angry and assign blame for mistakes of the past. As you read this book, please keep in mind that we cannot go back. We can only remain stuck where we are now or go forward.

While this book is written to Americans, its message also applies to the remaining 7 billion human beings on Planet Earth. It is the hope of this li'l old fat lady that there will be a few who will be able to raise themselves above the ideas of the time. I hope there will be a few who will be able to turn the kaleidoscope and be able see what *can* be rather than what *is*.

Following are two examples of how our understanding of things has changed over time. Example two also shows how long it can take for a few to be able to raise themselves above the ideas of the time.

EXAMPLE ONE

1822—Standard 1822 *medical textbook* regarding the cause of yellow fever.
"…[It] rises from the exposure of putrid animal and vegetable substances on the public wharfs…it always begins in the lowest part of a populous mercantile town near the water, and continues here without much affecting the higher parts. It rages most where large quantities of new ground have been made by banking out the rivers for the purpose of constructing wharfs…the yellow fever is generated by the impure air or vapour which issues from the new-made earth or ground raised on the muddy and filthy bottom of rivers…."[1]

2012—Wikipedia description of the cause of yellow fever.
(It's not necessary to read the entire Wikipedia article, but it shows we know a lot more today about yellow fever than we did in 1822.)

"The yellow fever virus is mainly transmitted through the bite of the yellow fever mosquito *Aedes aegypti*, but other mosquitoes such as the 'tiger mosquito' (*Aedes albopictus*) can also serve as a vector for the virus. Like other Arboviruses which are transmitted via mosquitoes, the yellow fever virus is taken up by a female mosquito which sucks the blood of an infected person. Viruses reach the stomach of the mosquito, and if the virus concentration is high enough, the virions can infect epithelial cells and replicate there. From there they reach the haemocoel (the blood system of mosquitoes) and from there the salivary glands. When the mosquito sucks blood the next time, it injects its saliva into the wound, and thus the virus reaches the blood of the bitten person. There are also indications for transovarial and transstadial transmission of the yellow fever virus within *A. aegypti*, i.e., the transmission from a female mosquito to her eggs and then larvae. This infection of vectors without a previous blood meal seems to play a role in single, sudden breakouts of the disease. There are three epidemiologically different infectious cycles, in which the virus is transmitted from mosquitoes to humans or other primates. In the urban cycle, only the yellow fever mosquito *Aedes aegypti* is involved, which is well adapted to urban centres and can also transmit other diseases including Dengue and Chikungunya. The urban cycle is responsible for the major outbreaks of yellow fever that occur in Africa. Except in an outbreak in 1999 in Bolivia, this urban cycle no longer exists in South America and is only present in Africa.

Besides the urban cycle there is, both in Africa and South America, a sylvatic cycle (Forest cycle or Jungle cycle), where *Aedes africanus* (in Africa) or mosquitoes of the genus *Haemagogus* and *Sabethes* (in South America) serve as a vector. In the jungle, mainly non-human primates get infected; the disease is mostly asymptomatic in African primates. In South America, the sylvatic cycle is currently the only way humans can infect themselves, which explains the low incidence of yellow fever cases on this continent. People who become infected in the jungle can carry the virus to urban centres, where *Aedes aegypti* acts as a vector. It is because of this sylvatic cycle that yellow fever cannot be eradicated.

In Africa there is a third infectious cycle, also known as savannah cycle or intermediate cycle, which occurs between the jungle and urban cycle. Different mosquitoes of the genus *Aedes* are involved. In recent years this is the most common form of yellow fever seen in Africa."[2]

EXAMPLE TWO

1973—Dr. Robert C. Atkins was vilified and labeled a fraud by the American Medical Association, the United States government, and the press for daring to suggest that carbohydrates make us fat.

1977—History of American diet doctrine from the book *Good Calories, Bad Calories,* by Gary Taubes.

> By 1977, when the notion that dietary fat causes heart disease began its transformation from speculative hypothesis to nutritional dogma, no compelling new scientific evidence had been published. What had changed was the public attitude toward the subject. Belief in saturated fat and cholesterol as killers achieved a kind of critical mass when an anti-fat, anti-meat movement evolved independent of the science.[3]

> [On] January 14, 1977, Senator George McGovern announced the publication of the first *Dietary Goals for the United States.* The document was "the first comprehensive statement by any branch of the Federal Government on risk factors in the American diet," said McGovern… Goal number one was to raise the consumption of carbohydrates until they constituted 55–60 percent of the calories consumed. Goal number two was to decrease fat consumption from approximately 40 percent, then the national average, to 30 percent of all calories, of which no more than a third should come from saturated fats.[4]

2010—From the SCIENTIFIC AMERICAN April 27, 2010.

> Eat less saturated fat: that has been the take-home message from the U.S. government for the past 30 years. But while Americans have dutifully reduced the percentage of daily calories from saturated fat since 1970, the obesity rate during that time has more than doubled, diabetes has tripled, and heart disease is still the country's biggest killer. Now a spate of new research, including a meta-analysis of nearly two dozen studies, suggests a reason why: investigators may have picked the wrong culprit. Processed carbohydrates, which many Americans eat today in place of fat, may increase the risk of obesity, diabetes and heart disease more than fat does—a finding that has serious implications for new dietary guidelines expected this year….Will the more recent thinking on fats and carbs be reflected in the 2010 federal Dietary Guidelines for Americans, updated once every five years?[5]

The answer is *no*. The US Department of Agriculture continues to recommend the old dietary dogma that has made Americans so overweight and obese, with the rates of diabetes, heart disease, and more increasing every day. And our United States government continues to blame the American consumer for the obesity epidemic. It's obviously all our fault because we're just not eating right. Here are the guidelines.

"The USDA Dietary Guidelines for Americans, 2010, released on January 31, 2011, emphasize three major goals for Americans:
- Balance calories with physical activity to manage weight
- Consume more of certain foods and nutrients such as fruits, vegetables, whole grains, fat-free and low-fat dairy products, and seafood
- Consume fewer foods with sodium(salt), saturated fats, *trans* fats, cholesterol, added sugars, and refined grains"[6]

2012—More than two hundred million Americans are now overweight or obese, and the rates of diabetes and heart disease are still skyrocketing. But, beginning in 2004, this li'l old fat lady defied all three 2010 USDA Dietary Guidelines. I raised myself above the ideas of the time to lose 90 pounds without dieting and send diabetes and heart disease scurrying in defeat. Because I got fed up and defied current diet doctrine, I regained my personal freedom and health. I have my cake and eat it too.

PART I

WHAT'S WRONG AND SOME DIETARY FIXES

CHAPTER 1

Just a Li'l Old Fat Lady Who Got Fed Up

The definition of insanity is doing the same thing over and over again and expecting different results.—Albert Einstein

Let me introduce myself. My name is Peggy June Forney and I'm a 61-year-old, 5-foot-3-inch-tall woman who got fed up with our current diet doctrine. So, I went from being extremely obese and sick to normal weight and healthy. And I did it without dieting. No calorie counting and no fat restrictions. Lots of rich, baked pastries, fried chicken, ice cream, pizza, eggs, bacon, chocolate, cheese, and butter. Let me say it again—I did not diet.

It took a long time, but 90 pounds slowly melted off. To give you some idea of what 90 pounds is, here is a list of clothes sizes I went through. First there were the Women's sizes 22, 20, 18, 16, and 14, then the Misses sizes 16, 14, 12, and 10. Most of my clothes are now Misses size 8. That's 10 sizes.

Let me tell you what else I lost. Diabetes and heart disease also went scurrying in defeat. While this may sound too good to be true, it really did happen. By defying current diet doctrine, I was able to regain both my personal freedom and my health. And if I can do this, just about anyone can do it. There are very few overweight or obese folks out there who would not achieve the same or better results than I did.

No, I'm not a "health professional" with lots of suffixes behind my name. There are already plenty of those out there claiming to know it all regarding your weight and health issues. Nope, I'm just a li'l old (formerly) fat lady who lost 90 pounds without dieting and who regained her health and freedom. I also have a special aptitude and a professional marketing track record for looking at lots of unrelated facts and then coming up with out-of-the-box solutions. But let me start at the beginning.

The first time I became concerned about my weight, I was 12 years old. So I've been dealing with the weight issue for almost 50 years. Until I turned 42 and had a total hysterectomy, I was generally a normal weight, but I was always dieting. Weight Watchers, Nutrisystem, Slim-Fast—you name it, I tried it. I would initially lose weight, but the result was only temporary and I always gained back the weight I lost. The dieting process was really miserable. I was always hungry and crabby, but I thought I was just a weak-willed wimp.

However, it turns out that most people who diet don't achieve significant long-term weight loss. Here's what Lawrence Gould, an analyst at Datamonitor (an independent research company in the United Kingdom) says: "In 2002, 230.6 million people across Europe attempted a diet. Of these, only 3.8 million will succeed in keeping off the weight that they have lost for over a year."[1] When you do the math, that's only 1.6 people out of 100. The remaining 98.4% will fail. Why am I quoting a UK statistic instead of a US statistic? Because there doesn't seem to be an equivalent number that's widely available to the general public in the United States. I wasn't able to do a Google search and find this kind of information, and it doesn't appear to be posted on any of our US government websites.

The Federal Trade Commission (FTC) is the government agency that is charged with protecting you and me from scams and frauds. The FTC has a web page titled "Who Cares." Under the section, "Who Cares About Weight Loss Promises?" they've posted a list of five agencies who care about weight loss promises. Here's the list: FTC (ftc.gov/health), National Institute of Diabetes and Digestive and Kidney Diseases Weight-Control Information Network (win.niddk.nih.gov), Centers for Disease Control Division of Nutrition, Physical Activity, and Obesity (cdc.gov/nccdphp/dnpa), USDA Center for Nutrition Policy and Promotion (mypyramid.gov), and American Dietetic Association (eatright.org).[2]

Now, I'm sure all of these agencies do care about weight loss promises, but I can't seem to find any weight loss programs that actually make any weight loss promises. Let's take a recent Weight Watchers TV ad as an example. The glamorous Jennifer Hudson doesn't actually promise anything. She just sings, "Because It Works." Then we've got NBA Hall of Famer Charles Barkley with the "Lose Like a Man" campaign. Finally, there's the press release in which Weight Watchers proclaims 2012 "The Year to Believe."[3] None of these Weight Watchers statements make *any* promise of weight loss. That didn't stop US

News, in January 2012, from ranking Weight Watchers as the number one weight loss diet: "The best diet for losing weight is Weight Watchers."[4]

I did find an April 18, 2000, MedscapeWire article that references a letter. The letter was written to Dr. Allen M. Spiegel, director of the NIDDK (National Institute of Diabetes and Digestive and Kidney Diseases), by a coalition of prominent academic researchers and authors of best-selling diet books. The letter states, "The debate will not end—and overweight people will not have reliable information to guide their attempts to lose weight until well-designed independent research investigates the effectiveness of different approaches."

This same MedscapeWire article also states that Dr. George Blackburn, associate professor of nutrition and surgery at Harvard Medical School, also urged Congress to call on the NIH (National Institutes of Health) to sponsor research on obesity. "For 30 years, Americans have been trying every sort of weight-loss diet imaginable, but there is precious little research on the safety and effectiveness of any of them. Because NIH hasn't sponsored the research on its own, Congress should insist it do so."[5] I went to the NIH website but couldn't find any research that documented long-term weight loss program metrics. But, in the 12 years since the coalition letter and Dr. Blackburn's appeal to Congress, overweight and obesity rates have gone from 64% in 1999–2000[6] to 68.5% in 2007–2010.[7]

I also went to the big national weight loss companies' websites and looked for the long-term weight loss metrics associated with each program. Unfortunately, I came up empty handed. I'm not the only one.

Here's what CBS News has to say about a recent review published in a 2009 *Annals of Internal Medicine* (American College of Physicians):

> **Diet Plan Success Tough to Weigh.**— A review of 10 of the nation's most popular weight-loss programs found that, except for Weight Watchers, none of them offer proof that they actually work at helping people shed pounds and keep them off. Only Weight Watchers had strong documentation that it worked—with one study showing that participants lost around 5% (about ten pounds) of their initial weight in six months and kept off about half of it [five pounds] two years later.[8]

With its five-pounds-two–years-later weight loss results, Weight Watchers does as well as any of the weight loss programs. The graph below is a five-year weight loss chart from a study conducted by the American Society for Clinical Nutrition titled *Long-term weight-loss maintenance: a meta-analysis of US Studies* that analyzed results from 29 weight loss studies.[9] The title of the graph is "Weight reduction maintained over time." Even though the graph is a little hard to read, what's not hard to read is that most people who lose weight will regain a substantial amount. At year one, weight loss ranged from approximately six kilograms to 17 kilograms (13–37 pounds). At year five, the average (triangle) weight loss appears to be just over two kilograms, or approximately five to six pounds. Based on this study, Weight Watchers' results and my own long-term weight loss program experiences are right on the money. At least for the US weight loss industry, estimated at $62 billion annually.[10]

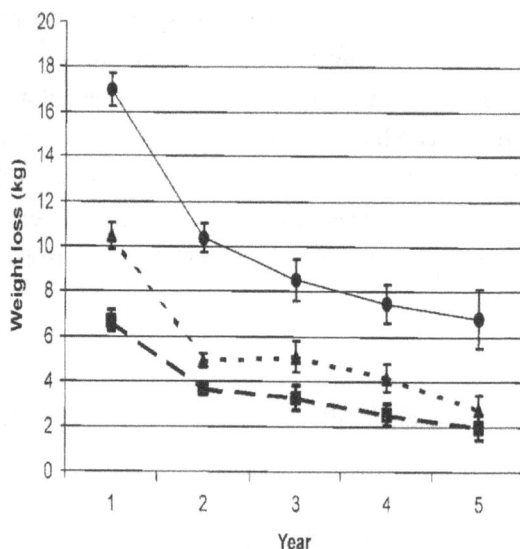

11

OK, let's get back to how I got so obese and then lost 90 pounds and regained my personal freedom and health. After the hysterectomy, I lost control. My weight steadily increased until it topped the 230-pound mark, which put me in the BMI (Body Mass Index) category of "Extreme Obesity." According to the BMI charts, I should weigh 107–140 pounds.[12] By the time I turned 52, I was diagnosed with "insulin resistance" (a physiological condition where the natural hormone insulin becomes less effective at lowering blood sugars),[13] which means that I was well on my way to becoming a type 2 diabetic, and my high cholesterol levels required prescription Lipitor. At this point, I was taking multiple prescription medications for my rapidly deteriorating health.

While I was extremely obese, it became difficult to do everyday things that normal-weight people take for granted. Climbing stairs would leave me completely breathless and drained. I would seek out the handicapped bathroom stalls because they had more room. I was always hot, and I couldn't do any sort of physical activity without being in complete misery. Even personal hygiene became a challenge. I could not move freely, so I had lost my personal freedom as well as my health.

One day in early 2004, a TV news program featured the CDC (Centers for Disease Control). I don't remember what the topic was, but I did remember the CDC. A few weeks later, I was surfing the net and the CDC was featured again. This time I clicked on the link and followed that link to another link and another link and so on. I ended up on a page that showed obesity rates by age group. The obesity rates for each age group steadily increased until age 65-plus, which was the oldest age group listed. The obesity rate for the 65-plus age group was about half of the younger age groups.

I still remember how terrified I felt when I saw the number. That number was tiny because *fat people do not live to be old people. And the diseases fat people die of are not pleasant.* I am not afraid of dying, but I am desperately afraid of needles. And I knew that I would be experiencing lots of needles and pain because I was obese and sick. Why did that single number have such a traumatic impact on me? The answer to this question goes back to a test I took in high school.

While I was in high school, my entire class was required to take some sort of IQ/aptitude test. School always required tests, so I didn't pay any attention, especially since I wasn't working for a grade. A day or two later I got called to the principal's office. Now, getting called to the principal's office was generally never a good thing. Although I didn't know what I had done, I was still worried. It turned out I was called because the principal and the people who had administered the test just wanted to ask me some questions. They told me the test results for one section of the test were completely skewed and they were trying to figure out why. As I remember back 40-plus years, my test scores were extraordinarily high in one area, but all of the other test scores were just average. My test scores didn't make any sense to the principal or the testers, and that's why they wanted to talk to me. At the time, I shrugged off their puzzlement—I was just relieved because I wasn't in trouble.

Over the decades I've learned that my brain is both a gift and a curse. It's a gift because I can see new things differently from many people, but it's a curse because I have great difficulty figuring out how to communicate in a way that helps others see what I see.

Because of my unusual brain, I see the world of facts sort of like a kaleidoscope. The number of colors and patterns are almost endless and, as you turn the tube, they all change. My brain processes information much like a kaleidoscope. It takes lots of little bits of unrelated information and forms a completely new and different picture out of the bits and pieces.

So when I saw the CDC number I panicked. Based on that single number, my kaleidoscope brain immediately saw a myriad of implications associated with the number. Age 65-plus fat people were not dieting, but dying, thus leaving only the thin ones to be counted. On average, *fat people do not live to be old people. And the diseases that were killing the fat people were horrible.* They were not dying peacefully in their sleep. There was lots of suffering before they died. As an extremely obese person, this was my future. I did not want to experience this future, so I needed to become normal weight. The question was, how?

The answer to this question had been provided by Dr. Eric Leder, MD, my primary care physician of more than 25 years. Approximately 10 years earlier, I had been trying to lose a few pounds by using Slim-Fast. One of my office coworkers needed to lose 20 pounds from being pregnant, and she thrived on Slim-Fast. Boy, did she look good! So, I substituted Slim-Fast for breakfast and lunch and the pounds began to come off.

Then, I began to feel sick. Like the flu sick. I felt a little better in the mornings, so I would go to work, but the afternoons were horrible. I finally made an appointment with Dr. Leder because something was definitely wrong. Dr. Leder reminds me of the recently deceased actor Peter Falk in the TV series *Columbo* because he is amiable and doesn't try to impress folks with fancy furniture and decorator art. You might have a tendency to underestimate him, but he is a brilliant detective and will eventually come up with the correct answer. Like Columbo, he always gets the villain, and that's why he's been my physician for more than 25 years.

So I went in with my strange flulike symptoms, and Dr. Leder patiently listened and asked lots of questions. After I got done rambling on and on and he had poked and prodded, he finally pronounced his diagnosis. It was "reactive hypoglycemia caused by the Slim-Fast." He said he thought the Slim-Fast contained too much sugar for my particular digestive system. (Slim-Fast currently offers a Lower Carb Vanilla Cream shake and a Lower Carb Creamy Chocolate shake.)[14] I was so shocked that you could have picked me up off the floor. How could I be making myself feel so sick when one of my coworker friends felt so good?

Dr. Leder told me that he could put me through a long, multiple-hour, glucose toler-ance testing process with multiple blood draws (horrible needles!), or I could simply follow the instructions he gave me on a single piece of paper. If his diagnosis was cor-rect, he said I would feel much better within two weeks. The sheet had two columns of food items. One column was all the foods that I could eat, and the other column contained all the foods I was supposed to avoid. I remember looking at the sheet of paper and thinking that I would become as fat as a pig if I ate the "OK" list foods. That list contained lots of calories, fat, protein, and fiber. The "no-no" list contained wheat, rice, corn, potatoes, sugars, alcohol, and caffeine. Dr. Leder explained that he believed that my pancreas was ultrasensitive to quickly digested foods and that it produced too much insulin in response. The extra insulin quickly resulted in low blood sugar, which is why I felt like I had the flu.

I had a lot of respect for Dr. Leder, so I decided to try his solution. It was going to be difficult to stay away from many of the foods I loved, and I remember whining about giving up my coffee. Dr. Leder told me that the objective was to avoid stimulating my pancreas and, like sugar and carbohydrates, caffeinated coffee and alcohol did just that. When he saw my agonized look, he relented a little and told me to drink decaf coffee as much as possible.

Dr. Leder was right, and within two weeks I felt like my old energetic self. During this time, I couldn't bear to think about my weight, so I just ignored the scales. Then I had to go somewhere that required me to wear my jeans, and I dreaded putting them on. I knew they would be too tight. When I put my jeans on, they just hung on me. They were too big! For the second time in two weeks, I was totally shocked. How could this be? I had not been on a diet. As a matter of fact, many of the foods I had been eating were extremely high in calories and fat. So I stepped on the scales and discovered that my weight had dropped by six pounds. It just didn't make any sense. As time went on, I went back to eating foods on both lists, but I never forgot the mystery of my unexpected weight loss. It was the only time in my life that I had lost weight without dieting.

So when the CDC posted the ugly truth of what to expect as an extremely obese person, I decided to take what I had learned from Dr. Leder and implement it on a larger scale. I already knew that dieting had never worked for me in the past, so I decided this strat-egy of changing what I ate versus restricting how much I ate just might pay off. Because of my kaleidoscope brain, I saw a connection between the "OK" foods and my ability to lose weight. I was desperate, so I decided to take the gamble of turning myself into a human guinea pig.

Turns out, I went down a path that was often advocated by medical professionals and scientists prior to the low-fat, low-calorie, low-cholesterol craze that has helped make Americans obese. But I didn't know that. I just knew everything out there blared "diet" and that dieting had never worked for me in the past. It wasn't until I began researching for this book that I realized how much had been written since I began my weight loss journey in 2004. I will be referencing some of these books, and I strongly recommend you take the time and energy to read them.

The first author I'm going to recommend is Gary Taubes. Two of the books he's written are *Good Calories, Bad Calories*[15] and *Why We Get Fat.*[16] Taubes's *Good Calories, Bad Calories* book offers a fascinating accounting of the science and politics of how we Americans evolved into our current obesity crisis. The sequence of events during which America implemented the current dogma of low fat, low calorie, and low cholesterol is almost breathtaking. Gary actually pinpoints the day of the low-fat craze to Friday, January 14, 1977. That was the day that Senator George McGovern announced the publication of the first *Dietary Goals for the United States.*[17] This book leaves no stone unturned, but its 468 pages will exhaust you. To get started, I recommend you read Gary's other book, *Why We Get Fat*. It's only 225 pages and not nearly as heavy. Here's a short excerpt:

> *This is not a diet book, because it's not a diet we're discussing. Once you accept the fact that carbohydrates—not overeating, or a sedentary life— will make you fat, then the idea of "going on a diet" to lose weight, or what the health experts would call a "dietary treatment for obesity," no longer holds any real meaning. Now the only subjects worth discussing are how best to avoid the carbohydrates responsible—the refined grains, the starches, and the sugars—and what else we might do to maximize the benefits to our health.[18]*

So, back to me stumbling around in the dark back in 2004. I went ahead and implemented my plan of eating what I wanted, how much I wanted, and when I wanted, as long as it was on Dr. Leder's "OK" list. But it was definitely hard to stay away from all the foods that were on the "no-no" list. As time went on, I could see that I was going to have problems making this way of eating permanent, because I had given up so many of the wonderful foods that I had grown up with. So I became obsessed with finding really good substitutes for as many of the "no-no" foods as possible. Basically, I wanted to have my cake and eat it too.

But this book is not just about me losing 90 pounds and becoming healthy. It is about changing the way we think about diet and dieting. It's about changing the way we think about exercise. It challenges some of our current beliefs that have such a profound impact on the quality of our lives and our health. Even where we choose to live can make a difference. But most humans don't respond well to changing their beliefs. And many big businesses will feel threatened because fundamental change will require them to evolve their business models.

Because I know there will be some naysayers, it took a lot of courage and soul searching for me to decide to write this book. But it is a book that I believe should be written. The majority of Americans have lost a little or a lot of their personal freedom to be healthy and move freely. Using the latest CDC statistics from 2007 to 2010, a tragic 68.5% of adult Americans are now overweight or obese.[19] Using 2010 Census data,[20] that means that 150-million-plus adult Americans over the age of 20 are overweight or obese. And that obscene number doesn't include the growing epidemic of millions of overweight and obese children and adolescents. According to the American Heart Association, "Today, about one in three American kids and teens is overweight or obese, nearly triple the rate in 1963."[21] Using 2010 Census data, this means that more than 70 million young Americans are overweight or obese.[22] When you do the math, there are 200-million-plus overweight and obese Americans.

During an era of calorie counting and fat restriction, all we have done is become fatter and fatter. We've also become much less healthy, so health care costs are skyrocketing. According to the CDC, the medical care costs of obesity in the United States are staggering. In 2008 dollars, these costs totaled about $147 billion.[23] A new Cornell University study reports a figure of $190.2 billion per year and higher medical costs per obese person of $2,741.[24] In addition, an analysis of cost data from several major national databases confirms that the cost of managing the cardiovascular risks associated with obesity increase with the severity of the obesity. The analysis found that the cardiovascular risk factors of patients with a BMI over 35 cost health care payers an average of about $3,600 per person.[25] If these numbers aren't big enough, how about $861 billion to $957 billion by 2030? This is what the American Heart Association is projecting if the current trends in the growth of obesity continue.[26] That's a lot of money. Wouldn't it be nice to free this huge sum up for something else a little more pleasant and fun?

The brilliant Einstein said it best: *"The definition of insanity is doing the same thing over and over again and expecting different results."* Our current diet doctrine of counting calories and restricting fats is insane, and it's time for a change.

In each of the following chapters, I will present stories and quotes to help illustrate the concept I am trying to convey. These may initially appear to be unrelated to the goals of this book, and some of them are downright tacky and tasteless. But they each contain an important lesson that can help you turn the kaleidoscope to see beyond our current diet doctrine. Each story or quote can help you raise yourself above the ideas of the time.

You will also see an occasional "*Peggy Prediction.*" Here is one.

Peggy Prediction—*If every overweight or obese person in the United States eliminated PSS-rich foods from their diet, it would only take five years to virtually eliminate the obesity epidemic in this country.* **This prediction is explained and covered in detail in chapter 3.**

None of the dietary information I present in this book is original. The basic tenets have been advocated by medical professionals, scientists, and nutritionists for many decades. All I have done is translate some of their knowledge into li'l old fat lady language. The medical professionals, scientists, and nutritionists are the experts when it comes to this field, but they haven't persuaded the average overweight or obese person to actually change his or her eating habits. They haven't persuaded the processed food industry to change either. But maybe this li'l old fat lady might be able help.

Why do I think I'm qualified to help? Because I've learned how to lose 90 pounds and regain my health without dieting. I'm also a veteran marketing professional who has a stellar track record for getting folks to adopt and embrace "fundamental change." In the technology world, this type of change is called a Discontinuous Innovation, but the same rules also apply here. In 1986 I was verbally attacked for implementing a Discontinuous Innovation. But after I got over my initial shock, I became fascinated with this marketing specialty and spent the next 15 years focused on mastering the art and science of getting folks to adopt fundamental change. The strategies I offer in this book reflect those 15 years of learning from the school-of-hard-knocks. Later on, in chapter 10, I will present a more complete explanation of the Discontinuous Innovation concept.

There is one tool that you will need as you read this book. It is a large, well-lit mirror. As you read this book, you may occasionally feel yourself becoming indignant about those guilty, greedy food processors and fast food joints that have created this unfortunate situation. If you do, you need to go look in the mirror. You and I are the consumers. You and I are in charge.

To those companies that I mention by name, you are just examples. All of us are in the same boat. If you see statements that make you angry and fearful, that's the goal of this book. We all need to get angry and fearful about our current obesity epidemic in this country. I had to get fed up before I could permanently lose 90 pounds along with regaining my health and freedom. Why? Because fundamental change never occurs unless there is serious discomfort with the current situation.

Finally, although this book recommends tearing apart some of our dearly held beliefs and changing our dietary strategies, this is a book of hope. It doesn't just tell you what is wrong; it also offers some realistic solutions. Solutions that allow you to have your cake and eat it too. Solutions that have the potential to make some American businesses a whole lot of money. But it requires changing our thinking and behavior. Change is never comfortable, but the survival of every species is dependent upon coping with it. This li'l old fat lady believes that the long-term economic survival of the United States of America is also at stake.

As I've stated before, this book is about fundamental change. It's about changing the way we look at our personal freedom. The freedom to eat what we want, when we want. The freedom to move freely. The freedom of being healthy. By raising ourselves above the ideas of the time, we can each regain our personal freedom and health.

Although the foundation is what we eat, there are other things that can help stack the deck in our favor. These things include physical activity and coping with friends and family who still think the earth is at the center of the universe. Even geography can play a role. By paying attention to all of these things, we can improve our chances of regaining our health and personal freedom.

So, I divided this book into four parts. Part I explains what's wrong and some dietary fixes. Part II focuses on additional things that can increase our chances of regaining our health and personal freedom. Part III provides foods, recipes, and pearls of wisdom from some nutritional experts. And Part IV offers some li'l old fat lady marketing strategies to help Americans get out of this terrible obesity and disease predicament.

Finally, fundamental change is always destructive. Fire is terribly destructive, but it ultimately allows new life to thrive. My goal is to provide out-of-the-box thinking and solutions that can help Americans do more in the way of controlled burns rather than deal with raging wildfires. The goal is to keep the pain of fundamental change to a minimum while moving Americans toward regaining our personal freedom.

In 1982, the major telecommunications company I worked for was split up by the government. Many of the long-time employees were traumatized because, instead of one big national company, there were suddenly going to be lots of smaller regional companies. As a coping tool, they gave each of the managers a little plastic cube. The purpose of the cube was to try and get the long-time employees to change their focus from looking at the trauma aspect of fundamental change to instead looking at the new opportunities that this fundamental change would offer. Even today, I still keep this little plastic cube on my desk and hope you will keep its message in mind for the remainder of this book. Yes, change does cause trauma, but it also creates new opportunities. Here's a picture of my little plastic cube.

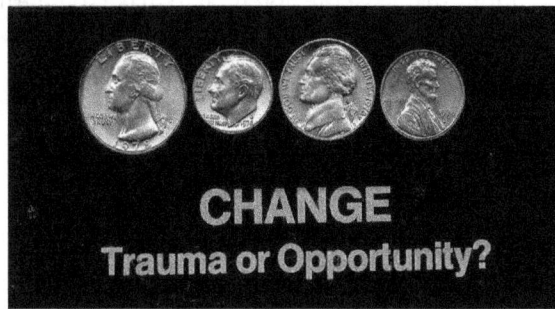

When you read this book, you may be tempted to ask why we can't just go back to the way things used to be. We can't. We can only move forward from where we are now. With over 7 *billion* human beings living on this planet, we can't go back. We can only work to make our current situation better. Yes, we *can* make our current situation better, but we need to embrace rather than resist fundamental change. Resisting fundamental change will only make our long-term prospects even worse.

There's a bicycle manufacturer named Specialized.[27] Like Trek, Giant, and others, they make really good bicycles. You know, the type that Lance Armstrong rides. These high-end bicycle companies are in head-to-head competition to be the best bicycle manufacturer out there. They are dealing with a moving target because, every year, if they don't produce the very best product in the market, someone else will. Each of these high-end bicycle manufacturers is constantly seeking new materials and new ways to produce a better, higher-performing bicycle. Schwinn used to be the leader in this market, but they became comfortable and complacent. So they lost their place as the head of the pack.

Specialized is the company that introduced the "Stumpjumper," the first mountain bike, over 30 years ago. Even today, mountain bikes are still a major consumer product. Throughout the decades, Specialized has continued to be an innovator in this industry and has not backed away from their company motto, *"Innovate or Die."* [28] I adopted the Specialized *"Innovate or Die"* motto during my weight loss journey. It worked for me and it can work for you. This is the culture that all Americans need to adopt so we can regain our personal freedom and health. Focusing on the Specialized *"Innovate or Die"* motto can help you raise yourself above the ideas of the time.

This li'l old fat lady also hopes that many big businesses will adopt the Specialized *"Innovate or Die"* motto and change their focus from protecting their current market position to seizing this new and exciting opportunity for unprecedented growth and profits. Yes, there *is* a way for big business to make big money. But we all need to see what *can* be rather than what *is*. We must all raise ourselves above the ideas of the time.

CHAPTER 2

Earth is *Not* at the Center of the Universe

All great truths begin as blasphemies.
—George Bernard Shaw (1856–1950)

Galileo (1564–1642) was an Italian physicist, mathematician, astronomer, and philosopher who played a major role in the scientific revolution. Up until the time of Galileo, it was believed that the earth was at the center of the universe. Because of his stance that the sun, not the earth, was at the center of the universe, Galileo was ordered to stand trial on suspicion of heresy in 1633. He was placed under house arrest for the rest of his life.[1]

Of course, we now know that Galileo was correct. But he was punished for trying to change the current thinking on the subject, and history is full of these examples. The process of changing people's thinking is always traumatic, painful, and lengthy.

This li'l old fat lady believes our current thinking on calories, fat, and cholesterol is as wrong as thinking that the earth is at the center of the universe. But, we've all grown up this way, so what we've been told just seems right to us. Let's take the calorie. What is a calorie? What does a calorie measure? Until about 120 years ago, the calorie concept didn't even exist. Here is my favorite definition of a calorie from www.theofficediet.com:

> Calories measure energy, particularly heat energy. One calorie is the energy required to raise the temperature of one gram of water by one degree Celsius. Nowadays, the calorie is only used for food energy—it's considered archaic in other contexts.[2]

In my opinion, the calorie concept is archaic in *all* contexts, *especially* when it comes to food. What does raising the temperature of water have to do with human nutrition? Nothing! Now, please don't send me to jail on suspicion of heresy. We're supposed to have the right to freedom of speech in America. Here's a little calorie counting history from Jonny Bowden, PhD, CNS, in his book, *Living Low Carb.*

> In 1917…an L.A. physician named Dr. Lulu Hunt Peters published what had to be the first calorie-counting book ever, *Diet and Health, with Key to the Calories.* She sold 2 million books, making it the first best-selling diet book in America. And here's the thing: by making calorie-counting equivalent to weight control, she also injected her own view of morality into the equation. People who couldn't control their calories (and therefore their weight) just lacked self-discipline. We can thank Dr. Peters for popularizing the concept that being overweight is a sign of moral weakness.[3]

So, eating lots of calories will make you fat. Right? And eating fat will make you fat. Right? And eating cholesterol will make your cholesterol levels go up and clog your arteries to give you heart disease. Right? That's not what happened to me as I lost 90 pounds. I ate all the calories, fat, and cholesterol I wanted, and my weight and cholesterol levels all went down to normal. Type 2 diabetes retreated in defeat. I no longer need to take Lipitor (for high cholesterol levels) or any of the other prescription medications that I needed to take when I was extremely obese. And, according to Dr. Leder, I am now completely healthy in all respects. So something else has got to be going on, or maybe I'm just special. I've been accused of that when people see what I eat.

Here is a typical breakfast for me: two butter-fried eggs, two sausage links, and a nice, rich piece of homemade raspberry cream cheese coffee cake. The number of calories, fat, and cholesterol in this breakfast are obscene according to current diet doctrine. But, that's what I ate as I lost 90 pounds. That's how I will continue to eat. Does this sound like dieting to you?

To avoid being burned at the stake for violating every current nutritional tenet in the universe, maybe it's time for a little Nutrition 101 discussion. In 1971, I took a two-unit college class in nutrition and I remember studying a thing called the Krebs cycle. It's also known by several other terms, such as the citric acid cycle, etc. Turns out, the concept is still regarded as current in the scientific community.

Since I'm just a li'l old fat lady, maybe I can get away with quoting stuff from Wikipedia. I selected Wikipedia because it is a nonprofit organization and does not depend financially upon funding and advertising from big business or big government. Wikipedia also doesn't use quite as much scientific-ese as some of the other sources I looked at, and I thought us regular folks might go cross-eyed if the vernacular got too thick. But don't let the simple, precise explanations fool you into thinking that the scientific community isn't on the same page.

Here's what Wikipedia has to say about the Krebs cycle:

> The Krebs cycle is a series of enzyme-catalyzed chemical reactions, which is of central importance in all living cells, especially those that use oxygen as part of cellular respiration….In aerobic organisms [humans], the Krebs cycle is part of a metabolic pathway involved in the chemical conversion of **carbohydrates, fats** and **proteins** into carbon dioxide and water to generate a form of usable energy. [**Peggy's Comment** - *Maybe I'm just blind, but I'm not seeing the word "calorie."*]

> [Regarding proteins]…proteins are essential parts of organisms and participate in virtually every process within cells. Many proteins are enzymes that catalyze biochemical reactions and are vital to metabolism. Proteins also have structural or mechanical functions, such as actin and myosin in muscle and the proteins in the cytoskeleton, which form a system of scaffolding that maintains cell shape. Other proteins are important in cell signaling, immune responses, cell adhesion, and the cell cycle. Proteins are also necessary in animals' [including humans'] diets, since animals cannot synthesize all the [20] amino acids they need and must obtain [9] essential amino acids from food. Through the process of digestion, animals break down ingested protein into free amino acids that are then used in metabolism. [**Peggy's Comment** - *Basically, you need to eat good quality proteins that contain the 9 essential amino acids or your health will suffer and you could possibly even die.*]

> [Regarding fats,] Vitamins A, D, E, and K are fat-soluble, meaning they can only be digested, absorbed, and transported in conjunction with fats. Fats are also sources of essential fatty acids, an important dietary requirement. Fats play a vital role in maintaining healthy skin and hair,

insulating body organs against shock, maintaining body temperature, and promoting healthy cell function.

Fats also serve as energy stores for the body, containing about 37.8 kilojoules (9 calories) per gram of fat. They are broken down in the body to release glycerol and free fatty acids. The glycerol can be converted to glucose by the liver and thus used as a source of energy.

Fat also serves as a useful buffer towards a host of diseases. When a particular substance, whether chemical or biotic—reaches unsafe levels in the bloodstream, the body can effectively dilute—or at least maintain equilibrium of—the offending substances by storing it in new fat tissue. This helps to protect vital organs, until such time as the offending substances can be metabolized and/or removed from the body by such means as excretion, urination, accidental or intentional bloodletting, sebum excretion, and hair growth.

While it is nearly impossible to remove fat completely from the diet, it would also be unhealthy to do so. Some fatty acids [omega 3 and omega 6] are essential nutrients, meaning that they can't be produced in the body from other compounds and need to be consumed in small amounts. All other fats required by the body are non-essential and can be produced in the body from other compounds. [**Peggy's Comment** - *The fat we're trying so hard to avoid actually plays a critical role in our overall health. So, let's see how much of it we can remove from our foods.*]

Foods high in carbohydrate include fruits, sweets, soft drinks, breads, pastas, beans, potatoes, bran, rice, and cereals. Carbohydrates are a common source of energy in living organisms; however, no carbohydrate is an essential nutrient in humans. Carbohydrates are not necessary building blocks of other molecules, and the body can obtain all its energy from protein and fats.[4] [**Peggy's Comment** - *The body can obtain all its energy from protein and fats. We don't need to eat carbohydrates to live. But the FDA tells us we should scarf down 300-375 grams of the stuff each day.*]

Peggy Prediction: *For the past 35 years, the US government's dietary guidelines have been emphasizing carbohydrates at the expense of proteins and fats. Fix this imbalance and you'll fix the obesity epidemic. Fix the obesity epidemic and you'll fix runaway diabetes, heart disease, and much more.*

Let's pause here for a moment and examine what I just stated. In 2009, 2010, and 2011, the National Center for Chronic Disease Prevention and Health Promotion Division of Nutrition, Physical Activity, and Obesity (breath), which is part of the CDC, published a four-page booklet titled *Obesity: Halting the Epidemic by Making Health Easier.*[5] This CDC booklet states, "The causes of obesity in the United States are complex and numerous, and they occur at social, economic, environmental, and individual levels." The booklet goes on and on about funding 25 states to work with partners across multiple settings and strategies to address the five target areas identified by the CDC for preventing and reducing obesity. Unfortunately, I just can't seem to find "making health easier" anywhere in this CDC booklet.

So, here's this li'l old fat lady's version of "making health easier." The causes of obesity are not complex and numerous. There is only one cause and it's not complex. It's excessive carbohydrate consumption. Period. This li'l old fat lady is living proof. Now that's easy!

OK, back to what we eat. Since proteins and fats are essential to keep us alive, let's pause here and take a closer look. First, we need to eat foods that contain the nine essential amino acids. Here's what Wikipedia has to say:

> A *complete protein* (or *whole protein*) is a source of protein that contains an adequate proportion of all nine of the essential amino acids necessary for the dietary needs of humans or other animals. Some incomplete protein sources may contain all essential amino acids, but a complete protein contains them in correct proportions for supporting biological functions in the human body.

The following table lists the optimal profile of the essential amino acids, which comprises a complete protein:

Essential Amino Acid	mg/g of Protein
Tryptophan	7
Threonine	27
Isoleucine	25
Leucine	55
Lysine	51
Methionine + Cystine	25
Phenylalanine + Tyrosine	47
Valine	32
Histidine	18

Nearly all foods contain all 20 amino acids in some quantity. However, proportions vary, and some foods are deficient in one or more of the essential amino acids. Apart from some exceptions such as quinoa or soybeans, vegetable sources of protein are more often lower in one or more essential amino acids than animal sources, especially lysine, and to a lesser extent methionine and threonine.

Generally, proteins derived from animal foods (meats, fish, poultry, cheese, eggs, yogurt, and milk) are complete, though gelatin is an exception. Proteins derived from plant foods (legumes, grains, and vegetables) tend to be limited in essential amino acids. Some are notably low, such as corn protein, which is low in lysine and tryptophan.[6]

Here is what Wikipedia has to say about essential fatty acids:

> *Essential fatty acids*, or *EFAs*, are fatty acids that humans and other animals must ingest because the body requires them for good health but cannot synthesize them. The term "essential fatty acid" refers to fatty acids required for biological processes, and not those that only act as fuel.
>
> Only two EFAs are known for humans: alpha-linolenic acid (an omega-3 fatty acid) and linoleic acid (an omega-6 fatty acid). Other fatty acids that are only "conditionally essential" include gamma-linolenic acid (an omega-6 fatty acid), lauric acid (a saturated fatty acid), and palmitoleic acid (a monounsaturated fatty acid).[7]

Maybe Wikipedia just isn't "expert" enough. Well, then, how about a medical doctor's opinion? Dr. Richard K. Bernstein, MD, is an expert on diabetes and has written several books, including *The Diabetes Solution*[8] and *The Diabetes Diet*.[9] Here's what Dr. Bernstein has to say: *"There are essential amino acids and essential fatty acids, but there is no such thing as an essential carbohydrate."*[10]

Now, let's review the 2010 USDA Dietary Guidelines against the science. The USDA says, *"Consume more of certain foods and nutrients such as fruits, vegetables, whole grains, fat-free and low-fat dairy products, and seafood."*[11]

Fruits, vegetables, and whole grains are high in nonessential carbohydrates and low in both essential proteins and essential fats, so the USDA says to eat more of them. And then, the USDA tells us to strip the essential fats out of our dairy products. But let's not be completely negative. The USDA did get it right regarding seafood. *Here's the bottom line. The USDA is telling Americans to emphasize a diet that largely contradicts the science.*

I want to stress that I'm not a medical professional, scientist, or nutritionist, so my expertise in this area is limited. But there are lots of really good books out there, including one called *Living Low Carb*, by Jonny Bowden, PhD, CNS.[12] This book does a good job of laying out the facts, and it critiques most of the major low-carb diets out there. There is also author Jimmy Moore with his two inspirational books, *Livin' La Vida Low-Carb*[13] and *21 Life Lessons from Livin' La Vida Low-Carb*.[14]

And there's a new book, *The Art and Science of Low Carbohydrate Living*, by Stephen D. Phinney, MD, PhD, and Jeff S. Volek, PhD, RD.[15] Now, if you want to get down and dirty and roll in the latest nutritional scientific-ese available, you will want to read this book. I'm not exaggerating—this book is guaranteed to make your eyes cross because it's written primarily for the scientific community. Read it and you'll have the latest medical/scientific information out there. It's also an excellent reference for doctors, nutritionists, and registered dietitians who want to learn how the sun is actually at the center of the universe. Don't believe this li'l old fat lady? Here's what weight loss expert doctor Michael R. Eades, MD, states on his blog: "I'm going to tell you about the best low-carb book I've ever read."[16] Now, I want to point out something that all of these books have in common. All of the titles contain versions of the phrase "Living Low Carb." The focus is not on dieting, but on living.

Now back to Jonny Bowden. He and I appear to disagree about calories. He says they do count, and I say they don't. I think we're both right. In his book, *Living Low Carb*, Jonny validly points out, "If I take in 15,000 calories all from fat with a little protein, producing the absolute minimum amount of insulin, I'm *still* going to gain weight."[17] He's right and I agree. But I'm saying that I lost 90 pounds by focusing solely on eliminating the excess carbohydrates from my diet. How could this work? Because, when I allow myself to eat good, rich foods that contain lots of protein and fat, my body just sort of turns on the brakes all by itself. My tendency to overeat evaporates. It's almost magic! And, it's is not just this li'l old fat lady's opinion. Here's what Dr. Richard K. Bernstein, MD, has to say in his book *Dr. Bernstein's Diabetes Solution*.

> …Most Americans who are obese are overweight not because of dietary fat, but because of excessive dietary carbohydrate. Much of this obesity is due to "pigging out" on carbohydrate-rich snack foods or junk foods, or even on supposedly healthy foods like whole grain bread and pasta. It is my belief that this pigging out has little to do with hunger and nothing at all to do with being a pig….I'm convinced that people who crave carbohydrate have inherited this problem. To some extent, we all have a natural craving for carbohydrate—it makes us feel good. The more people overeat carbohydrates, the more they will become obese, even if they exercise a lot. But certain people have a natural, overwhelming desire for carbohydrate that doesn't correlate to hunger. These people in all likelihood have a genetic predisposition toward carbohydrate craving, as well as a genetic predisposition toward insulin resistance and diabetes…This craving can be reduced for

many by eliminating such foods from the diet and embarking upon a low-carbohydrate diet.[18]

One of the "fundamental-change-hysterical-fear-routine" criticisms of Dr. Atkins's low-carbohydrate diet was the "dangers" of eating too much protein. In this book, when you see references to eating a high-protein, high-fat diet, it simply means eating a diet that emphasizes proteins and fats over carbohydrates. Here is what Jeff. S. Volek, PhD, RD, and Stephen D. Phinney, MD, PhD, say in their book, *The Art and Science of Low Carbohydrate Living.*

> As for how much is too much protein, this…has not been precisely defined. As a general rule, in the short term, people start to feel "unwell" if they routinely eat more than 30% of their daily energy need as protein. Even though low carbohydrate diets are often casually identified as high protein, the truth is most may not actually be that high. One factor driving this misunderstanding is that "protein foods" like bacon, eggs, fried chicken, tuna salad, hamburger, and even lean steak typically contain more fat calories than protein calories. So I fact, "high protein" diets consisting of common foods tend to be higher in fat than protein.[19]

And here's a quote from another book that you may also want to consider reading. The authors are talking about what happens when you eat excessive amounts of high-carbohydrate foods for decades. The book is titled *The New Atkins for a New You*, and the authors are Eric C. Westman, MD, Stephen D. Phinney, MD, PhD, and Jeff S. Volek, PhD, RD.

> This whole process is pretty silent for most of us, as long as we're young and healthy, but some people have trouble with these wide swings in blood glucose. If your insulin response is too great or lasts too long, your blood sugar level drops—and bam! your energy level crashes. You may recognize it as a slump a few hours after lunch. You may have trouble concentrating, feel sleepy, and often crave something such as chocolate, chips, or candy. Then guess what happens a few hours later. Just rerun the tape. Keep up this pattern for years, and you may develop insulin resistance, meaning that more and more insulin is required to transport the same amount of glucose. What has happened is that your body is giving in to the bully and the stage is set for developing metabolic syndrome and even type 2 diabetes.[20]

As a child I remember seeing exactly what these authors are describing. My mother had the same carbohydrate sensitivity I do, and the older she got, the more she suffered. She became extremely obese and couldn't lose weight. She did finally lose weight, but it wasn't until she was dying during the final stages of terminal breast cancer that had metastasized into her blood and bones.

An acquaintance of mine has repeatedly tried to get me to see the error of my ways. As a matter of fact, there have been times when this acquaintance has become downright mean. I guess losing 90 pounds and becoming completely healthy just isn't good enough. This individual is highly educated and very intelligent, but here are his precise words: "You need to eat sugar for your brain."

Let's follow his flawed logic to its ridiculous conclusion. The Inuit Eskimos of the Arctic have been extensively studied because their native diet consists almost solely of meat and fat. The researchers who studied the Inuit Eskimos reported that they had virtually no heart disease, cancer, or obesity. Now, these Eskimos lived in very cold harsh weather conditions and hunted and fished to stay alive and actually thrive. But they must have been the biggest morons on earth because they didn't feed their brains any sugar.

This is the kind of thinking that has caused the current obesity epidemic in this country. And this acquaintance isn't the only one. Here is a label from a Chiquita banana.

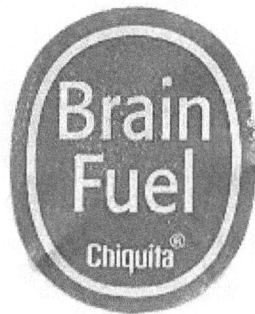

Back to the Inuit Eskimos. Perhaps these Eskimos were special humans unlike the rest of us? I've been accused of the same thing when people see what I eat. Gary Taubes' book *Good Calories, Bad Calories* offers a fascinating description of Harvard anthropologist-turned-Arctic-explorer Vilhjalmur Stefansson, who spent a decade eating nothing but meat among the Inuit of northern Canada and Alaska. Here are some excerpts from Taubes's book.

In the winter of 1928, Stefansson and Karsten Anderson, a thirty-eight-year-old Danish explorer, became the subjects in a yearlong experiment that was intended to settle the meat-diet controversy. The experiment was planned and supervised by a committee of a dozen respected nutritionists, anthropologists, and physicians...The only dramatic part of the study was the surprisingly undramatic nature of the findings...Both men were in good physical condition at the end of the observation ...There was no subjective or objective evidence of any loss of physical or mental vigor.

None of Stefansson's observations would have been controversial had not the conventional wisdom at the time been—as it is still—that a varied diet is essential for good health. A healthy diet, it is said must contain protein, fats, and carbohydrates, the latter because of the misconception that the brain and central nervous system require *dietary* glucose to function, and the debatable assumption that fresh vegetables and fruit, which contain carbohydrates, are essential to prevent deficiency diseases.

Because it is still common to assume that a meat-rich, plant-poor diet will result in nutritional deficiencies, it's worth pausing to investigate this issue. The assumption dates to the early decades of the twentieth century, the golden era of research on vitamins and vitamin-deficiency diseases, as one disease after another—scurvy, pellagra, beriberi, rickets, anemia—was found to be caused by a lack of essential vitamins and minerals...This philosophy, however, was based almost exclusively on studies of deficiency diseases, all of which were induced by diets high in refined carbohydrates and low in meat, fish, eggs, and dairy products.

What the nutritionists of the 1920s and 1930s didn't then know is that animal foods contain all of the [9] essential amino acids (the basic structural building blocks of proteins), and they do so in the ratios that maximize their utility to humans. They also contain twelve of the thirteen essential vitamins in large quantities. Meat is a particularly concentrated source of vitamins A, E, and the entire complex of B vitamins. Vitamins D and B12 are found only in animal products (although we can usually get sufficient vitamin D from the effect of sunlight on our skin).[21]

Pages 320–326 of *Good Calories, Bad Calories* completely rip apart the balanced diet dogma that has continued to blind us to the underlying dietary truths. It's a real eye opener, and as I read this part of Gary's book, I experienced anger because I too had been misled for so many decades. As I stated before, *Good Calories, Bad Calories* is very heavy reading, but Gary Taubes leaves no stone unturned. If you want to truly understand how Americans have become so obese and ill, I suggest you read this book.

Finally, more than any other book, *Good Calorie, Bad Calories* also illuminates a fundamental issue that has plagued some of the best scientific minds for the past 100 years. Although there are many brilliant researchers, scientists, medical doctors, nutritionists, and authors who have clearly articulated pristine nutritional enlightenment facts and data, the old, outdated dietary dogma and thinking still thrives. History is repeating itself. It's the "Galileo Effect" all over again—only the details are different. To repeat Voltaire, *Every man is the creature of the age in which he lives; very few are able to raise themselves above the ideas of the time.*

As of 2012, America has 200-million-plus people who are overweight or obese, and the number continues to increase every day. Diabetes, hypertension, cancer, heart disease, Alzheimer's disease, and more continue on their upward march. Simultaneously, the American economy continues on its downward spiral.

So perhaps now is a good time to change the terms of engagement. Maybe changing the rules can help Americans understand that the earth is not at the center of the universe. Later on in this book, this li'l old fat lady with the kaleidoscope brain will offer an out-of-the-box solution that can change the rules without forcing a single American to change his or her thinking or behavior.

CHAPTER 3
The *Real* Bad Boy on the Block

Hindsight is 20/20.—English Aphorism

Nat Geo Wild recently ran a TV program featuring the strange behavior of sea lions on the beaches around Monterey Bay, California, in the 1998–2000 time frame. The sea lions suffered from seizures and disorientation, and MRIs of the sea lions' brains revealed that they had suffered brain damage. More than 400 sea lions died during this tragic event. In analyzing the contents of the sea lions' stomachs, the researchers found traces of domoic acid. Turns out that the domoic acid came from anchovies that the sea lions ate. The anchovies ate algae blooms that occur every spring in the coastal waters. Normally, the algae blooms are benign and actually kick-start and feed the entire marine food chain. But, for some strange reason, the algae began producing poisonous domoic acid, which was ingested by the anchovies.

The anchovies that ate the algae weren't poisoned, because the domoic acid got stored in their bile. But the sea lions weren't that lucky, so it looks like the culprit must be the poisonous algae. Right? Well, not so fast. Why do normally benign algae suddenly start producing domoic acid that's poisonous? That was a real stumper for the researchers.

Fortunately, there were some really smart scientists involved, and they did a very good job of communicating with each other. Someone noticed that the poisonings occurred during El Niño. El Niño is a weather phenomenon that produces higher than normal temperatures and lots of rain. The researchers figured out that the excess rainwater running off the land into Monterey Bay contained higher than average concentrations of urea during the time of the sea lion poisonings. Urea is a widely used, benign substance that we humans put into all sorts of stuff, ranging from cosmetics to fertilizer.

The scientists figured out that higher than average concentrations of urea caused the algae to begin producing poisonous domoic acid, which caused the anchovies to become poisonous to the sea lions. While a modest amount of urea is perfectly normal in nature, we humans were the culprits who tipped the balance and made something toxic happen. The sea lions were the innocent victims.

The same phenomenon is occurring in the American diet. There's an imbalance that's causing more and more of us to get fatter and unhealthier. While we've been obsessed with demonizing calories, fats, and cholesterol, the *real* bad boy on the block just smiles. We're told that if we would just eat healthier and get more exercise, our problems would go away. If we wouldn't eat like gluttons and biggie-size everything at the fast food joints, we would be normal weight. We're told we fat folks are just weak-willed wimps and we're bad, bad, bad.

The minorities and less educated must be badder and worser than the whites because they're fatter. Women are fatter than men, so they must be badder and worser, too. Right? It must be so, because that's what the CDC's numbers are showing. Right?

Well, this li'l old fat lady says *wrong*! I believe we have been fixated on calories, fats, and cholesterol while the *real* bad boy on the block continues to cause all sorts of problems. Like the poor maligned algae that produced the poison that killed the sea lions, the real issue is that we Americans have created a carbohydrate imbalance in our food supply. I know we didn't do it on purpose. But it still happened, so maybe it's time to 'fess up and start working on fixing our predicament. It won't be painless, but the successful outcome will be absolutely wonderful.

Like the sea lions, the *real* bad boy on the block isn't easy to see. The problem involves multiple variables that play havoc when we're trying to figure out the riddle. Here's this li'l old fat lady's explanation of what's happening.

Going back to the Krebs cycle, we humans process proteins, fats, and carbohydrates into something that allows us to live. Everything we eat falls into one of those three buckets. And, just like everything else in nature, there is a delicate balance that needs to be maintained. We Americans have really screwed up this balance, and we're going to continue to suffer until we fix it. Right now, the number of Americans suffering is 200 million-plus and still rising.

To add to the confusion, we humans are not all exactly the same. So, we each react differently to this imbalance. Some of us appear to suffer more than others by becoming fat. You notice I say appear? I believe that most Americans are suffering from this imbalance, but it's just not as obvious for some folks. While a few people are not getting fat, they are still suffering negative consequences in more subtle and insidious ways. One negative consequence is hyperinsulinemia (high blood sugar).

Michael R. Eades, MD, and Mary Dan Eades, MD, are physicians who specialize in weight loss. In their book *Protein Power*, they use the term *normal weight, metabolically obese* and state that people who have never had a problem with excess weight have the most difficult time because any kind of food restriction has never been a part of their mind-set.[1] Yes, normal weight folks can and do suffer from hyperinsulinemia (high blood sugar), diabetes, elevated cholesterol, and high blood pressure.

Now, here's someone who writes from *normal weight, metabolically obese* personal experience. Author Jeff O'Connell's book, *Sugar Nation*, spells it out in exquisite detail. The catalysis for Jeff's book was the type 2 diabetes that killed his father and threatened Jeff's own life. Neither man was overweight. Here's a brief excerpt from Jeff's book describing his father.

> During my last visit, the stump remaining from his amputation had been covered; now it's exposed. The sight shouldn't surprise me, but I'm taken aback. His torso is covered with a polo shirt; his lower half, by a diaper. His remaining leg is propped up, and skinlike parchment flaps from the bone. His eyes widen when he sees me. Slowly, he extends an emaciated arm covered with blotches to hold my hand.[2]

At least the poor suffering man can still see. Diabetes is now the leading cause of new cases of blindness in America. While Jeff's father gets two painful catheters inserted into his arm for dialysis treatment because his kidneys don't work anymore, the two men have a final chance to talk. No, decades of excessive carbohydrate consumption doesn't just make us fat.

Jeff O'Connell is no lightweight. He is the editor-in-chief at Bodybuilding.com and previously served as executive writer at *Men's Health*, and editor-in-chief at *Muscle & Fitness*. Although *Sugar Nation* gets very graphic at times, it's a must read for anyone who's serious about regaining his or her personal freedom and health. Jeff's book helps explain why one in three US adults now has diabetes or prediabetes, and why many of us don't even know it. Before my 90 pound weight loss journey, I was one of them.

Just so you don't think that Jeff and I are being hysterical about diabetes, I have "cut and pasted" the actual wording from our federal government's NIH (National Institutes of Health) website. Here it is—read'm and weep.

Estimated Diabetes Costs in the United States, 2007

Total costs—direct and indirect	$174 billion
Direct medical costs	$116 billion—after adjusting for population age and sex differences, average medical expenditures among people with diagnosed diabetes were 2.3 times higher than what expenditures would be in the absence of diabetes
Indirect costs	$58 billion—disability, work loss, premature mortality

Medical expenses for people with diabetes are more than 2 times higher than for people without diabetes.

Complications of Diabetes in the United States

Heart Disease and Stroke
- In 2004, heart disease was noted on 68 percent of diabetes-related death certificates among people ages 65 years or older.
- In 2004, stroke was noted on 16 percent of diabetes-related death certificates among people ages 65 years or older.

- Adults with diabetes have heart disease death rates about 2 to 4 times higher than adults without diabetes.
- The risk for stroke is 2 to 4 times higher among people with diabetes.

Hypertension
- In 2005–2008, of adults ages 20 years or older with self-reported diabetes, 67 percent had blood pressure greater than or equal to 140/90 millimeters of mercury (mmHg) or used prescription medications for hypertension.

Blindness and Eye Problems
- Diabetes is the leading cause of new cases of blindness among adults ages 20–74 years.
- In 2005–2008, 4.2 million—28.5 percent—people with diabetes ages 40 years or older had diabetic retinopathy, and of these, 655,000—4.4 percent of those with diabetes—had advanced diabetic retinopathy that could lead to severe vision loss.

Kidney Disease
- Diabetes is the leading cause of kidney failure, accounting for 44 percent of all new cases of kidney failure in 2008.
- In 2008, 48,374 people with diabetes began treatment for end-stage kidney disease.
- In 2008, a total of 202,290 people with end-stage kidney disease due to diabetes were living on chronic dialysis or with a kidney transplant.

Nervous System Disease
- About 60 to 70 percent of people with diabetes have mild to severe forms of nervous system damage. The results of such damage include impaired sensation or pain in the feet or hands, slowed digestion of food in the stomach, carpal tunnel syndrome, erectile dysfunction, or other nerve problems.
- Almost 30 percent of people with diabetes ages 40 years or older have impaired sensation in the feet, for example, at least one area that lacks feeling.
- Severe forms of diabetic nerve disease are a major contributing cause of lower-extremity amputations.

Amputations
- More than 60 percent of nontraumatic lower-limb amputations occur in people with diabetes.
- In 2006, about 65,700 nontraumatic lower-limb amputations were performed in people with diabetes.

Dental Disease

- Periodontal, or gum, disease is more common in people with diabetes. Among young adults, those with diabetes have about twice the risk of those without diabetes.
- Adults ages 45 years or older with poorly controlled diabetes—A1C above 9 percent—were 2.9 times more likely to have severe periodontitis than those without diabetes. The likelihood was even greater—4.6 times—among smokers with poorly controlled diabetes.
- About one-third of people with diabetes have severe periodontal disease consisting of loss of attachment—5 millimeters or more—of the gums to the teeth.

Complications of Pregnancy

- Poorly controlled diabetes before conception and during the first trimester of pregnancy among women with type 1 diabetes can cause major birth defects in 5 to 10 percent of pregnancies and spontaneous abortions in 15 to 20 percent of pregnancies. On the other hand, for a woman with pre-existing diabetes, optimizing blood glucose levels before and during early pregnancy can reduce the risk of birth defects in their infants.
- Poorly controlled diabetes during the second and third trimesters of pregnancy can result in excessively large babies, posing a risk to both mother and child.

Other Complications

- Uncontrolled diabetes often leads to biochemical imbalances that can cause acute life-threatening events, such as diabetic ketoacidosis and hyperosmolar—nonketotic—coma.
- People with diabetes are more susceptible to many other illnesses. Once they acquire these illnesses, they often have worse prognoses. For example, they are more likely to die with pneumonia or influenza than people who do not have diabetes.
- People with diabetes ages 60 years or older are 2 to 3 times more likely to report an inability to walk one-quarter of a mile, climb stairs, or do housework compared with people without diabetes in the same age group.
- People with diabetes are twice as likely to have depression, which can complicate diabetes management, than people without diabetes. In addition, depression is associated with a 60 percent increased risk of developing type 2 diabetes.

Diagnosed and Undiagnosed Diabetes among People Ages 20 Years or Older, United States, 2010

Group	Number or percentage who have diabetes
Ages 20 years or older	25.6 million, or 11.3 percent, of all people in this age group
Ages 65 years or older	10.9 million, or 26.9 percent, of all people in this age group
Men	13.0 million, or 11.8 percent, of all men ages 20 years or older
Women	12.6 million, or 10.8 percent, of all women ages 20 years or older
Non-Hispanic whites	15.7 million, or 10.2 percent, of all non-Hispanic whites ages 20 years or older
Non-Hispanic blacks	4.9 million, or 18.7 percent, of all non-Hispanic blacks ages 20 years or older

Sufficient data are not available to estimate the total prevalence of diabetes—diagnosed and undiagnosed—for other U.S. racial/ethnic minority populations.

Diagnosed and Undiagnosed Diabetes

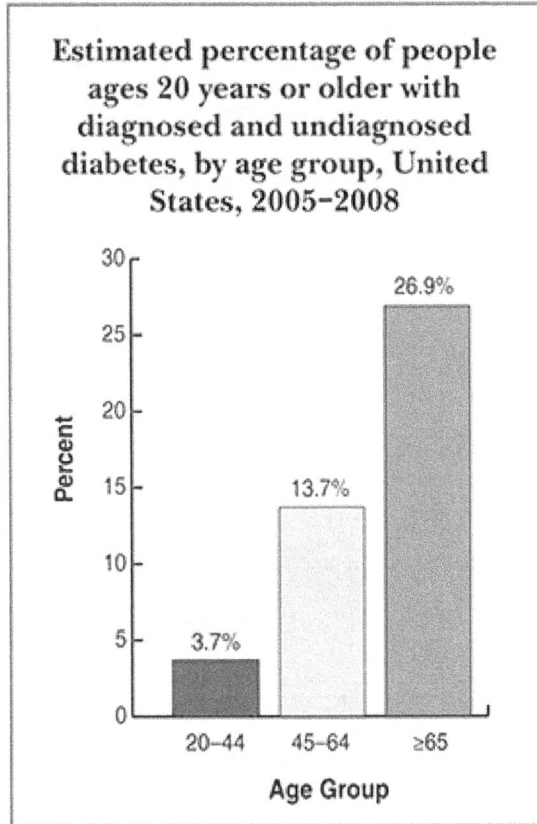

Estimated percentage of people ages 20 years or older with diagnosed and undiagnosed diabetes, by age group, United States, 2005–2008

26.9%

13.7%

3.7%

Percent

20–44   45–64   ≥65

Age Group

Source: 2005–2008 National Health and Nutrition Examination Survey

From the National Institute of Diabetes and Digestive and Kidney Diseases (NIDDK), National Institutes of Health (NIH).[3]

After what you've just read, you may feel like the best option you have is to slit your wrists. But we *can* triumph over this situation. Here's what Michael R. Eades, MD, and Mary Dan Eades, MD, say in their book *Protein Power*. They are speaking about reversing heart disease, which takes some time. This li'l old fat lady has found new 2012 scientific research that shows diet may significantly improve diabetes in as little as three days. The research is described later on in this chapter.

> Are we doomed to live with the current state of our coronary arteries barnacled with plaque, or can we reclaim them? We can reclaim them, but not overnight. The development of plaque takes time, and so does

its regression; it's a process that takes years, not months. It can also be done only in the face of a *lowered insulin level.*

In the words of one researcher, a consistent finding in animal studies is that insulin "inhibits regression of diet-induced experimental atherosclerosis, and insulin deficiency inhibits development of arterial lesions." In other words, if you want to clean up your coronary arteries, you can't do it in the presence of hyperinsulinemia. Unfortunately, when plaque has reached the point of calcium deposition, hemorrhage, and excess fibrous tissue formation, it is irreversible despite insulin lowering; even at that point, however, dietary intervention can forestall further formation.[4]

So we humans are actually better off than the poor brain-damaged sea lions—many of us still have time to turn our ship around. This is exactly what I did eight years ago. *By eliminating hyperinsulinemia before permanent damage was done, I sent diabetes and heart disease scurrying in retreat. I no longer suffer from either of these terrible diseases and was able to eliminate all of the prescription medications that were associated with them.*

Just like the urea example, it's important to realize that carbohydrates are not bad—it's the imbalance that's bad. Using the sea lion example of how an imbalance can cause benign algae to become toxic, I'm going to show you how an imbalance of carbohydrates in our diet can cause our pancreas to become toxic. The pancreas is a very special organ. Its role is to produce insulin, which is essential for us to live. Without insulin, we will die. But too much insulin will also kill us. It's that delicate balance thing. Here's what Michael R. Eades, MD, and Mary Dan Eades, MD, have to say in their book *Protein Power.*

Although it performs countless other tasks throughout the body, insulin's chief priority is to keep the blood sugar level from rising too high. Glucagon's main function is to prevent the blood sugar level from falling too low. The importance of this minute-by-minute regulation of the level of sugar in the blood is underscored by the fact that without either one of these hormones we would be dead in a matter of days or perhaps even hours.[5]

Up until about 100 years ago, we didn't have this blood sugar imbalance. Henry Ford hadn't introduced the Industrial Revolution, planes hadn't taken over the sky, and scientists hadn't played God with the genetics of all of our foods. But all that started changing in the early 1900s.

So, why don't we just turn back the hands of time and go back to the good old days? You know, the days of organic free-range chickens hunting and pecking in our rural yards and cows and sheep basking in the sunshine out in the pasture. The days of picking wild, organic raspberries and raiding bees' nests out in the wilderness. You know, those good old days. We can't go back, we can only move forward. Why? Well, it's got something to do with feeding seven *billion* human beings. Unless something really horrible and catastrophic happens to a large number of the humans on this planet, we just have to accept where we are now. But, we don't have to be content with letting the bad things stay bad. There are lots of things we can do to improve life on this planet—that's what this book is all about.

So, things are fine as long as we human beings don't muck with the delicate balance of Mother Nature, but we just can't seem to resist. And we don't have the ability to see what's going to happen until after it's happened—it's the old "hindsight is 20/20" rule. Then, we have to fix whatever it is that we screwed up.

Now, here's another li'l old fat lady with the kaleidoscope brain observation. This one is also about Mother Nature. We humans like to believe we're intelligent and rational. The distinctive red Nike swoosh and tag line "Just Do It" is a wonderful marketing strategy, and I applaud Nike. But "Just Do It" doesn't apply to eating. No animal does anything because it is good for it. Every animal does everything because it is pleasurable. Human beings are no exception. Mother Nature has a brilliant strategy of making pleasurable everything that is essential for our ongoing existence. Sex, eating, drinking water, sleeping, babies, relationships, you name it, it's pleasurable. Some of us human beings like to think we can outwit Mother Nature, but we're wrong. Here is what Robert H. Lustig, MD has to say.

> We love it. We go out of our way to find it. There is no food stuff on the planet that has fructose that is poisonous to you. It is all good. So, when you taste something that is sweet, it's an evolutionary Darwinian signal that this is a safe food. We were born this way.[6]

The next point is that we humans have a tendency to become addicted to things that stimulate the pleasure centers of our brain. Cocaine, smoking, and alcohol are well-known examples. We will seek these things out even when our intelligent, rational brain tells us that we are making a big mistake. Less well known is the addictive nature of excessive carbohydrates and sugars in "comfort foods" and sweet desserts. The taste of sweet causes our brains to emit dopamine and we experience pleasure. As long as we don't muck with Mother Nature, that's a good thing.

But Americans *have* mucked with Mother Nature, and we are producing foods that upset the delicate balance. The vast majority of what we take off of the grocery store shelves and put in our shopping carts contains added carbohydrates. And the "natural" carbohydrates like wheat, corn, potatoes, and rice have been bred, genetically modified, and processed so that they cause our pancreas to poison us. Ditto with many of our mainstream fruits and vegetables.

So we've become fixated on organic this and organic that to try and keep us healthy. Organic is a good thing, but it doesn't address the imbalance that we've created. Organic products typically cost 10% to 40% more than similar conventionally produced products.[7] So I believe the biggest thing organic has done is make some folks feel good about themselves and generate more income for the producers. If you don't believe me, here are the numbers. Organic really got rolling in the early 1990s with the world organic market growing by 20% a year.[8] Since 1990, the obesity rate in this country has gone from 12%[9] to 35.7% in 2009–2010,[10] along with huge increases in diabetes and heart disease. As I said before, organic is a good thing, but it isn't fixing our current obesity and health crisis in this country.

Back to the pancreas and the insulin it produces. As long as things are in balance, life is good. But the American diet screws this balance up. *The thing that stimulates the pancreas to produce insulin is carbohydrate.* Here's what the medical doctors and nutrition experts are saying.

> *A steady diet heavy in carbohydrates (such as the USDA Food Pyramid diet, which encourages consumption of carbohydrate foods equivalent to about 2 cups of sugar a day), necessitates a high, regular insulin output to handle all that incoming glucose. This constant demand on the system eventually takes its toll and the insulin receptors become less and less responsive to insulin's signal. This dulling of the receptors is termed "insulin resistance," which mountains of medical research have implicated as the root cause of the constellation of disorders known as the metabolic syndrome, or syndrome X. Among the disorders commonly associated with this syndrome are elevated cholesterol, low HDL cholesterol, high*

triglycerides, high blood pressure, diabetes, reflux and severe heartburn (gastroesophogeal reflux disorder, or GERD), sleep apnea, and central obesity."—Michael R. Eades, MD, and Mary Dan Eades, MD[11]

Whether you eat a piece of the nuttiest whole grain bread, drink a Coke, or have mashed potatoes, the effect on blood glucose levels is essentially the same—blood sugar rises, rapidly, and in proportion to carbohydrate content.—Richard K. Bernstein, MD[12]

The primary stimulator of insulin release from the pancreas is dietary carbohydrate. In contrast, an equal amount of dietary energy as fat has virtually no effect on insulin levels.—Jeff S. Volek, PhD, RD, and Stephen D. Phinney, MD, PhD[13]

So, fat consumption produces no insulin response and protein consumption produces modest insulin response.[14] As long as our consumption of carbohydrates is balanced as Mother Nature intended, everything is OK. But we Americans have created an obesity epidemic by putting too many carbohydrates on our plates and in our stomachs.

What about "natural" sweet fruits like that Chiquita banana? How could I possibly say bananas aren't good for us? I'm not saying they aren't good for us. But, in nature, bananas grow in limited geographic areas and aren't available 365 days a year. We humans have mucked with Mother Nature so that every grocery store in the nation has bananas available every day of the year. And when you add that banana to the top of the Kellogg's Corn Flakes and liberally sprinkle them with sugar and then add skim milk, you've dumped an incredible overdose of carbohydrates into your digestive system. Oh, don't forget that doughnut and the French Vanilla coffee sweetener. The inevitable result is a toxic pancreas.

Individual humans are each programmed to need more or fewer carbohydrates, depending on our genetic makeup. Just like fingerprints, we are all unique, and there is no one rule that will work for everyone. But if we're all eating too many carbohydrates, we're all going to have some sort of negative result.

Peggy Prediction: *We're eventually going to come to the realization that excessive carbohydrate consumption doesn't rot just teeth.*

Let's look at some quantitative stats about the direct link between excessive carbohydrate consumption and obesity and diabetes. Here's a 2004 *American Journal of Clinical Nutrition* study titled "Increased consumption of refined carbohydrates and the epidemic of type 2 diabetes in the United States: an ecological assessment." According to this study:

> In this ecologic analysis, in which national data from 1901 to 1997 were used, we found a strong association between an increased consumption of refined carbohydrates in the form of corn syrup, a decreased consumption of dietary fiber, and an increasing trend in the prevalence of type 2 diabetes in the United States during the 20th century. Furthermore, our data are consistent in that obesity and the prevalence of diabetes increased proportionately to the increase in consumption of refined carbohydrates in the United States.

> Our data also indicate that modern carbohydrates are considerably different from those consumed before the beginning of the 20th century and that the US food supply has become reliant on highly refined carbohydrates as significant sources of energy. The refining process has changed the composition and thus the quality of carbohydrates. For example, processing whole grains into white flour actually increases the caloric density by > 10%, reduces the amount of dietary fiber by 80%, and reduces the amount of dietary protein by almost 30%. Refining removes many of the main ingredients, leaving a dietary substance that is nearly pure starchy carbohydrate with fewer nutrients.[15]

Now here are some pictures to go with the stats. Following are two charts from this same study that quantify the link between decades of excessive carbohydrate consumption and obesity and diabetes in our country. Yes, it does take a while for the *real* bad boy on the block to show his ugly face.

OBESITY IN AMERICA

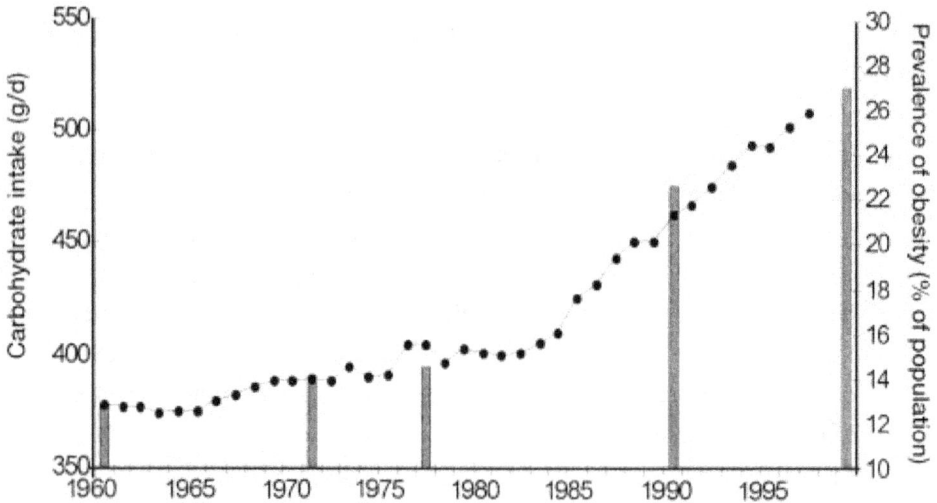

Figure 5. Increasing prevalence of obesity [BMI (in kg/m2) > 30; vertical bars] in the United States between 1960 and 1997 with increasing carbohydrate intake.[16]

DIABETES IN AMERICA

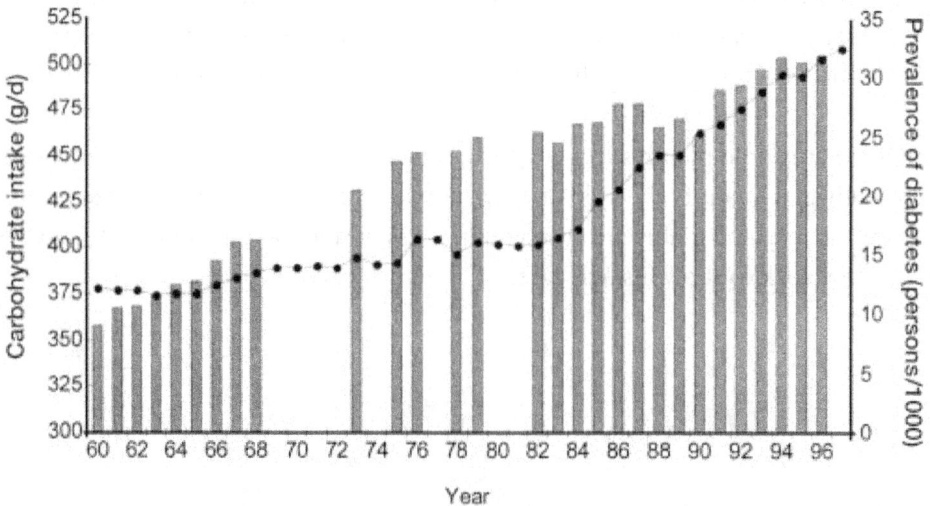

Figure 4. Increasing prevalence of type 2 diabetes (vertical bars) in the United States between 1960 and 1997 with increasing carbohydrate intake.[17]

OK, back to addictions. In the 1980s I was a "chain" coffee drinker. Basically, I drank caffeinated coffee all day. I don't remember why, but I decided that I wanted to quit drinking caffeinated coffee. I then developed a hideous headache and didn't feel especially good. One of my observant coworkers explained my predicament—caffeine withdrawal.

As we consume large quantities of certain substances, our amazing bodies compensate. We can consume more and more without feeling any different. But if we suddenly eliminate what we're consuming, the initial result is less than wonderful. The same is true for cocaine, tobacco, alcohol, and carbohydrates.

At first, we may feel the sensation of withdrawal. But when we get through that stage and then later try and go back to our original consumption levels, the result is just as dramatic. Many of us know what it is like to have an alcohol hangover. After not consuming alcohol for a while, just a little of the stuff will give you a nasty hangover. After not consuming excessive carbohydrates for an extended period of time, you get a similar hangover if you eat the same amount of carbohydrates that you used to eat.

Someone who consumes alcohol to the point of negative consequences is an alcoholic. For the most part, Americans are carboholics. We'll try and stay away from whatever our carbohydrate weakness is, but then we'll cave. We'll have a second helping and then another. We just can't seem to control ourselves. And we can't acknowledge that we're a carboholic. Is anyone looking in the mirror right now?

An acquaintance of mine suffers from high blood pressure and has suffered a TIA (mini stroke). He frantically restricts his salt intake, exercises like a maniac, is normal weight, and only buys healthy organic foods. Very proudly, he says he doesn't like sweets but then admits his weakness is salty snacks. The point he's missing is that, underneath the salt, there is an obscene amount of carbohydrates in all those organic snacks. If he kept track for a week of the total quantity of carbohydrates he was eating, he would be appalled. But I don't see that happening anytime soon.

Another acquaintance is even worse because she's trained as a medical professional and thinks she knows it all. What she knows is the current dietary dogma that has made so many Americans obese and sick. This acquaintance has been diagnosed with high cholesterol even though she's a health food nut, has a complete phobia of fat and animal protein, and exercises so much that she is slightly underweight. In the mornings she will eat a bowl of organic oatmeal for breakfast, but will avoid balancing it out with sufficient protein and fat. The result is a hypoglycemic "crash and burn" event sometime before lunch. Things get so bad that some of her friends actually carry extra snacks for her.

But carboholics are like alcoholics. They're so addicted they can't face the truth. Here's what a Bloomberg.com news article has to say.

> Cupcakes may be addictive, just like cocaine. A growing body of medical research at leading universities and government laboratories suggests that processed foods and sugary drinks made by the likes of PepsiCo Inc., and Kraft Foods, Inc. aren't simply unhealthy. They can hijack the brain in ways that resemble addictions to cocaine, nicotine and other drugs.

> "The data is so overwhelming the field has to accept it," said Nora Volkow, director of the National Institute on Drug Abuse. "We are finding tremendous overlap between drugs in the brain and food in the brain."

> The idea that food may be addictive was barely on scientists' radar a decade ago. Now that field is heating up. Lab studies have found sugary drinks and fatty foods can produce addictive behavior in animals. Brain scans of obese people and compulsive eaters, meanwhile, reveal disturbances in brain reward circuits similar to those experienced by drug abusers.

> Twenty-eight scientific studies and papers on food addiction have been published this year [2011], according to a National Library of Medicine database. As the evidence expands, the science of addiction could become a game changer for the $1 trillion food and beverage industries.

> If fatty foods and snacks and drinks sweetened with sugar and high fructose corn syrup are proven to be addictive, food companies may face the most drawn-out consumer safety battle since the anti-smoking movement took on the tobacco industry a generation ago.[18]

This li'l old fat lady believes that this article, while very illuminating, is actually throwing the baby out with the bath water. Fat has been the darling demon for so many decades in America that we just can't turn the kaleidoscope to see that carbohydrates are actually the *real* bad boy on the block. Fatty foods are not the culprit here. Turn off the carbohydrate spigot and fat will behave itself. Michael R. Eades, MD, and Mary Dan Eades, MD, say the same thing.

> When dietary fat and cholesterol do cause problems, it's usually *because* of the carbohydrate eaten along with them. It is true that fat is the raw material from which the body makes cholesterol, and it is also true that if you add more fat to your diet your cholesterol will increase, *but only if you continue to eat a lot of carbohydrate at the same time that you add the fat.*[19]

Peggy Prediction: *Based upon my own weight loss journey, I found it very easy to break the physical metabolic addiction to excessive sweets and carbohydrates. But, like alcoholism, nicotine, and other addictions, fixing the disturbances in my brain's reward circuits proved very difficult. So, I predict that after consuming excessive carbohydrates for many decades, the brain's abnormal, addicted desire for carbohydrates and the taste of sweets is almost impossible to break. That's why I have my cake and eat it too.*

Which brings me to another point. The word "carbohydrate" is a completely screwed-up term in America. The number of confusing words we apply to this element of the Krebs cycle is completely mind boggling. We've got the "good carbs" versus the "bad carbs," and the "natural sugars" versus the "artificial sweeteners." We've got the "simple sugars" versus the "complex carbohydrates." And we've got the "high glycemic index" foods versus the "low glycemic index" foods. The list just goes on and on. Here is what Richard K. Bernstein, MD, has to say about carbohydrates.

> So what are carbohydrates? The technical answer is that carbohydrates are chains of sugar molecules. The carbohydrates we eat are mostly chains of glucose molecules. The shorter the chain, the sweeter the taste. Some chains are longer and more complicated (hence, "simple" and "complex" carbohydrates), having many links and even branches. But simple or complex, carbohydrates are composed entirely of sugar. "Sugar?" you might ask, holding up a slice of coarse-ground, seven-grain bread. "This is sugar?" In a word, yes, at least after you digest it.[20]

Recently, the corn growers have been taking it on the chin. America has now decided that fructose (which the corn growers refer to as corn sugar) is the bad boy on the block, so we're hysterically running away from this bad boy. The corn growers don't like their shrinking profits, so the Corn Refiners Association has mounted a marketing campaign to try and convince us that they are actually good boys. Here's their campaign language, "Whether it's corn sugar or cane sugar, your body can't tell the difference. Sugar is sugar." Every time I see one of their TV ads, I laugh hysterically. I have to—it's either laugh or cry.

So, this li'l old fat lady came up with a new term for the *real* bad boy on the block. It's *PSS*[SM] which stands for *Pancreas Stimulating Substance*[SM]. Any and all foods that are not proteins or fats fall into this Krebs cycle category. This means there's no wiggle room for the *real* bad boy on the block. I've even come up with logos that identify the PSS content in foods, and you'll see them in chapter 9, "Foods and Recipes That Will Knock Your Socks and 90 Pounds Off," and in chapter 10, "Just One Fourth of a Penny." Like us humans, the shape of the logos changes from slim to fat as the PSS count increases. Here's a preview.

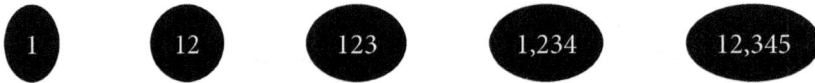

| 1 | 12 | 123 | 1,234 | 12,345 |

So when my physician Dr. Leder figured out what was wrong with me, his solution was to give my pancreas a break. Things like sugar, carbohydrates, alcohol, and caffeine all stimulate your pancreas to secrete insulin, so they were on the "no-no" list. Eliminating them from my diet for just two weeks made a huge improvement in how I felt. It also resulted in me losing six pounds even though I had increased my calorie and fat consumption. This is how I lost 90 pounds without dieting. This is how I regained my health. By using the term PSS, we include all of the bad boys and don't allow any of them to bob and weave around the issue.

Author Jimmy Moore has lost over 180 pounds by avoiding PSS-rich foods. His two inspirational books, *Livin La Vida Low-Carb* and *21 Life Lessons from Livin' La Vida Low-Carb*, document his successful journey from obesity and sickness to normal weight and good health. In *Livin' La Vida Low-Carb*, Jimmy refers to sugar as rat poison,[22] and I used to refer to sugar as arsenic. Over time, I've adjusted my thinking. Both rat poison and arsenic are known poisons. They don't hide in a dark closet. As a PSS, sugar and carbohydrates are worse. They are the *real* bad boys on the block precisely because they're not poisons. Similar to the sea lion example, excessive quantities of PSS make our magnificent pancreas slowly poison us to death by causing it to chronically emit too much insulin.

Peggy Prediction: *If every overweight or obese person in the United States eliminated PSS-rich foods from his or her diet, it would take only five years to virtually eliminate the obesity epidemic in this country.*

How did I come up with five years? Well, I figure an average weight loss of 150 pounds would go a long way towards eliminating the obesity epidemic. It took me three years to lose 90 pounds (average of 30 pounds per year) and I'm guessing that about 80–90% of the population would do better than me. Five years times 30 pounds results in 150 pounds of weight loss. Keep in mind that my expertise isn't math, but helping folks to adopt fundamental change.

So, what's the correct amount of PSS we should be consuming? The FDA Nutrition Facts labels on the processed food in my kitchen cabinets show 300 grams for someone consuming 2,000 calories per day and 375 grams for someone consuming 2,500 calories per day. The 112-page 2010 USDA Dietary Guidelines for Americans recommends that carbohydrates be 45–65% of total calorie consumption, and calorie consumption varies by age, gender, and activity level.[23] So, what's the recommended USDA number? There isn't one.

As a side note, since 1980, the USDA Dietary Guidelines have been issued every five years. Back in 1980, the guideline document was 11 pages long. Since that time, each edition of the document has increased in size to its current 112 pages.[24] So it fits right in with the 68.5% of Americans who have also become overweight or obese. OK, let's get back to the correct amount of PSS we should be consuming. The US Institute of Medicine recommends a minimum intake of 130 grams of carbohydrate per day.[25] And the *New Atkins for a New You* book recommends 20 grams per day and gradually increasing that number.[26]

Let's stop for just a moment and take a look back at Dr. Robert C. Atkins. While Dr. Atkins devoted his life to trying to keep us from the precise situation we're currently in, he was demonized by the American Medical Association (AMA), the press, and the United States government. Just like Galileo, who said that earth was not at the center of the universe, he was publicly denounced as a fraud. And, although it's tempting to cast blame on the AMA, press, and US government, this reaction is completely typical when humans are asked to accept fundamental change.

On April 12, 1973, Dr. Atkins testified before a Senate Select Committee on Nutrition and Human Needs Hearing and submitted a written statement for the record. Here are the introduction words that were made by Senator George McGovern, who presided over the committee: "The American Medical Association took the unusual step recently of publicly criticizing Dr. Atkins' diet recommendations as nutritionally unsound and potentially dangerous."[27] This is a perfect textbook example of the "fundamental-change-hysterical-fear routine."

The official record of this event can be obtained at www.hathitrust.org by searching under "nutrition and diseases 1973." I encourage you to read this almost-40-year-old document. It's quite shocking to see how much of what he predicted has turned out to be true. It will also quickly become clear that while Americans hold dear our right to freedom of religion and freedom of speech, the same does not hold true for freedom of diet. Even today, people who don't adopt a calorie- and fat-restricted diet doctrine can expect to be subjected to criticism, ridicule, and even hostility. But I'm sure it took just as long for some folks to accept that Earth was not at the center of the universe.

Back to the correct amount of PSS. Because we humans each have a unique metabolism, there is no one right number. Some of us are hypersensitive to PSS, so our threshold is very low. Other people can thrive on more PSS. Just like when the doctor asks you what your pain is on a scale of 1-10, with 1 being very little pain and 10 being complete agony, each of us must answer the question individually and subjectively. My own PSS threshold is very low. My subjective response is 2 on a scale from 1 to 10. While a few folks are more sensitive than me, I can tolerate very little PSS. At normal weight, I strive to keep my PSS consumption to an average of less than 40 grams a day. That means the daily total is less than one serving of regular pasta a day. That's about one tenth of the 375 grams of PSS (carbohydrates) recommended by the FDA for someone consuming 2,500 calories.

It's also less than one third of the average PSS intake of folks who think they are eating "low carb." During the low carb craze that occurred during 2003, CNNMoney.com reported, "A study of 11,000 people by market research firm NPD Group found that virtually none were cutting carbs to the degree that the low-carb diet recommends. Adults who have cut their carb intake are still eating about 128 grams of refined carbs a day on average—about 20 to 25 grams of carbs higher than a low-carb diet recommends for weight loss."[28]

In this li'l old fat lady's opinion, it's not because these 11,000 folks were weak-willed wimps, but partly because it was and still is impossible to just run down to your local grocery store or fast food joint and buy low PSS foods. It's also partly because we Americans didn't and still don't understand that decades of excessive PSS consumption will cause obesity, diabetes, heart disease, and hypertension, not to mention other afflictions that are starting to rear their ugly little heads. Things like complications from arthritis, metastasized cancer, and Alzheimer's disease, just to name a few.

Speaking of low PSS and normal weight, here's what I experienced as I went through my 90-pound weight loss journey. The first four months I lost approximately 24 pounds. That's an average of six pounds a month. At the end of the first 12 months, I was approximately 45 pounds lighter. That's an average of a little less than four pounds a month. The weight loss rate continued to slow and, after the first year, I relaxed my low PSS eating strategy. However, I never went back to eating PSS like I had done when I was obese. My weight loss stopped and my weight remained static for several years. But I did not regain the weight as I had done when I restricted calories and fats as a dieter.

After several years I decided that I needed to complete my weight loss journey, so I duplicated what I had done the first year and lost another 45 pounds. It took me two more years to achieve normal weight. Toward the end of my journey, the weight loss rate slowed to a trickle. Sometimes months would go by and the scales would not budge. Sometimes the scales would actually go in the wrong direction. So, on average, I lost about 30 pounds a year for three years. That's an average of two-and-a-half pounds a month. The good news is that the weight came off very rapidly at first and I quickly got much of my health and personal freedom back. The bad news is that I had to be very patient and tenacious at the tail end of the process.

Now, here's the most important point. I haven't changed my eating strategy at all even though I am now at normal weight. Nothing has changed. Even at normal weight, I am very PSS sensitive. That is why it is critical to adopt an eating strategy that you are willing to live with for the rest of your life. I'm completely happy with mine because I have my cake and eat it too.

In today's world of FedEx and G4 cellular technology, we always expect instant results. But while some desperate folks have even chosen gastric bypass surgery to try and save their health and regain their freedom, I'm not convinced that quicker is better. Here's why. By s-l-o-w-l-y losing the weight, you will allow your body to catch up with the new you. Now, the gastric surgeons who do the gastric bypass surgery and the plastic surgeons who cut off all the excess skin from the bodies of the newly thin will cringe, but the risk to the patient is considerable. Trust me, before they cut on you, they require you to sign all those surgical liability release documents for a reason.

While there's no rule that applies to every situation, this li'l old fat lady is not a fan of bariatric surgery. My dislike of bariatric surgery is based on what the scientists and researchers are saying, not on what big business is saying. So, let's take a close-up-and-personal look at bariatric surgery. Here is what the NIDDK (National Institute of Diabetes and Digestive and Kidney Diseases) has to say:

> Bariatric surgery restricts stomach size and/or leads to decreased absorption of nutrients. These procedures can have **significant** health benefits, such as reversal of type 2 diabetes or improvements in sleep apnea, but the procedures also carry substantial risks, including death.[2]

Now, according to the NIDDK, "bariatric surgery restricts stomach size and/or leads to *decreased absorption of nutrients.*" Remember the Krebs Cycle? What are the three components of human nutrition? They are carbohydrates, proteins, and fats. Although we may think this surgery just lowers our calorie consumption, it is actually preventing our body from absorbing the excessive PSS (carbohydrates) that are making us fat. *It also prevents our body from absorbing the essential proteins, essential fats, and other nutrients that help keep us alive and healthy.*

This is not just a li'l old fat lady's opinion. Here's what the NIDDK has to say about bariatric surgery:

> Examples of side effects that may occur later include nutrients being poorly absorbed, especially in patients who do not take their prescribed vitamins and minerals. In some cases, if patients do not address this problem promptly, diseases may occur, along with permanent damage to the nervous system. These diseases include pellagra (caused by lack of vitamin B3-niacin), beri beri (caused by lack of vitamin B1-thiamine) and kwashiorkor (caused by lack of protein).[30]

Now here's what the NIDDK has to say about our current weight loss strategies:

> Currently, the most effective way for people with extreme obesity to lose substantial amounts of weight and improve their weight-related health conditions is through bariatric surgery.
>
> Although an increasing number of persons with extreme obesity are undergoing bariatric surgical procedures, there has been little systematic

research to help determine its risks and benefits or to provide guidance on appropriate patient selection. To facilitate research in this area, NI-DDK established LABS (Longitudinal Assessment of Bariatric Surgery.)[31]

So, the NIDDK says our current best solution to treating the symptom of extreme obesity is to surgically restrict stomach size and *decrease our absorption of essential life giving nutrients.* How incredibly sad that the *real* bad boy on the block just smiles while desperate folks resort to life-threatening surgery.

Shockingly, this surgery doesn't guarantee permanent weight loss. According to a NIH study titled *Behavioral Predictors of Weight Regain After Bariatric Surgery,* "After bariatric surgery, a lifelong threat of weight regain remains." According to the study, 79% of the respondents reported some weight regain and 15% reported significant regain.[32] So, after undergoing risky bariatric surgery, most folks still don't have the freedom to eat what they want when they want. Nope, I think I'll just have my cake and eat it too. For the 79% of bariatric surgery patients who still have weight problems, take a look at chapter 9, "Foods and Recipes That Will Knock Your Socks and 90 Pounds Off."

Now here's a March 26, 2012, Associated Press headline, "Studies: Surgery can put diabetes into remission." The AP article states:

> New research gives clear proof that weight-loss surgery can reverse and possibly cure diabetes, and doctors say the operation should be offered sooner to more people with the disease—not just as a last resort...The results were dramatic: Some people were able to stop taking insulin as soon as three days after their operations. Cholesterol and other heart risk factors also greatly improved...There were signs that the surgery itself—not just weight loss—helps reverse diabetes. Food makes the gut produce hormones to spur insulin, so trimming away part of it surgically may affect those hormones, doctors believe...An obesity surgery equipment company sponsored the study, and some of the researchers are paid consultants; the federal government also contributed grant support.[33]

Let's review what the NIH says about bariatric surgery. "Bariatric surgery restricts stomach size and/or leads to decreased absorption of nutrients." So, here's this li'l old fat lady's interpretation of what these research findings may actually mean.

Peggy Prediction: *By simply changing dietary intake to restrict the excessive ingestion of diabetes- and heart-disease-causing carbohydrates, diabetic patients requiring insulin may be able to stop taking insulin in as soon as three days. Cholesterol and other heart risk factors will also greatly improve.*

The problem with this li'l old fat lady's interpretation of the research findings is that big business doesn't get to make big money. The surgeons, surgery equipment companies, hospitals, and paid consultants all lose out. Everybody in the bariatric surgery business loses, except the ill diabetic patient who is able to stop taking insulin and improve his or her health. So, this li'l old fat lady is willing to bet the study didn't include a control group of diabetic patients who ate a diet very low in carbohydrates but high in essential proteins and essential fats.

Now, there will definitely be some folks who question this li'l old fat lady's audacity. Fair enough. I'm not a medical doctor who specialized in diabetes. But Dr. Richard K. Bernstein, MD, *is* one of the foremost medical doctor experts on diabetes and its complications. His practice is solely devoted to diabetes and prediabetic conditions. He has also personally coped with type 1 diabetes for over 60 years, since he was 12 years old, and has followed a low carbohydrate diet since 1970. The introduction in Dr. Bernstein's 2005 book, *The Diabetes Diet*, reads, "How I Discovered the Low-Carbohydrate Diet and Saved My Own Life." The title of chapter 1 reads, "Why a Low-Carb Diet Is the Only Answer for Diabetics (and a very good answer for everyone else)."[34] So, that's why this li'l old fat lady would make such an "audacious" interpretation.

More and more of our precious little children are also going under the bariatric surgery knife. Here's a 2010 *Nature Publishing Group* article that makes my skin crawl, titled "Bariatric Surgery in Adolescents—The Sooner the Better?" The last sentence in the article states, "In conclusion, the increasing arsenal of bariatric procedures along with the development of novel anti-obesity pharmacological agents promise exciting options for the treatment of adolescents with morbid obesity in the future."[35] Yes, I would use the word "morbid."

And Magdalena Placka Östlund, MD, from the Karolinska Institutet in Stockholm, Sweden, reports that patients who undergo gastric bypass surgery have a twofold increased risk for inpatient treatment for alcohol abuse, compared with patients who have a restrictive procedure such as gastric banding. She said the association is most likely due to the altered metabolism of alcohol that occurs after gastric bypass. "A large portion of the stomach is bypassed and the alcohol passes straight to the small intestine and into the blood, where we see increased alcohol concentrations."[36] Ah, yes, let's put more drunk drivers on the road.

Finally, here's yet another little bariatric surgery hiccup. By six years after their surgery, people who have undergone bariatric surgery have a twofold chance of experiencing broken bones, especially in their hands and feet. Here's a statement from Jackie Clowes, MD, PhD, senior author of a study done by a research team from the Departments of Endocrinology, Health Sciences Research, and Rheumatology at the Mayo Clinic in Rochester, Minnesota. "We knew there was a dramatic and extensive turnover and loss of bone density after bariatric surgery. But we didn't know what that meant in terms of fractures."[37] Well, now we do. When you restrict the absorption of essential proteins and essential fats, you don't just lose weight.

Now, let's pause for a moment on the subject of bone density. When I was 56, after losing approximately 45 pounds by eating low PSS foods that were also high in essential proteins and essential fats, Dr. Leder casually suggested that I might want to consider getting a routine "baseline" bone density test. Although I didn't know this at the time, according to the NIH, "Women under age 65 are at increased risk for osteoporosis if they have early menopause [in my case, from surgery]."[38]

The medical facility I went to was brand new and the technician asked my permission to take a second set of pictures. They were putting together training materials and the technician wanted to include pictures of my bones because they "represent the ideal in bone density." So, at the ripe old age of 56, someone finally took beauty pictures of me. According to the NIH, "The T score compares your bone density with that of healthy young women…A T score is within the normal range if it is -1.0 or above…A T score between -1 and -2.5 indicates the beginning of bone loss (osteopenia)…A T score below -2.5 indicates osteoporosis."[39] So, while a score of -1.0 indicates normal bone density, *my* T score was *+1.6*.[40] Now, let's see—osteoporosis and broken bones or beauty pictures. Nope, I'll just stick with my cake and eat it too.

Peggy Prediction: *Bariatric surgery is a "canary in the mine" regarding osteoporosis. A high PSS diet that's low in essential proteins and essential fats will contribute to osteoporosis. A low PSS diet that's high in essential proteins and essential fats will help prevent osteoporosis.*

Bariatric surgery is also costly for the patient and the rest of us. According to the NIDDK, the average cost for bariatric surgery is $20,000-$25,000.[41] If there are any complications, the price tag can go as high as $69,960.[42] If there is an insurance company involved, that cost is passed directly on to all the rest of us in the form of huge insurance premiums that only keep going up. According to a Kaiser Family Foundation 2011 Annual Survey, the average 1999 annual insurance premium cost for family coverage was $5,845 (200-plus workers). The 2011 average annual insurance premium cost projection for family coverage was $15,520 (200-plus workers).[43] So the average annual insurance premium cost has nearly tripled in thirteen years. Let's not exaggerate. It's only 265% higher.

Now, according to the former American Society for Bariatric Surgery (now the American Society for Metabolic and Bariatric Surgery, or ASMBS), the estimate for bariatric surgeries in 2008 was 220,000.[44] So, 220,000 people got parts of their digestive systems surgically cut out or "banded," and we Americans paid between $5 billion and $8 billion just in 2008 just so we can keep our addiction to the *real* bad boy on the block.

Then there are the deaths from the surgery. According to the US Department of Health and Human Services, "The 6-month post-surgical death rate for patients operated on between 2005 and 2006 was 0.5%."[45] With more laparoscopic surgeries and other improvements, the NIDDK is now quoting a 0.3% death rate.[46] But, no one's really counting. Even the poor dead brain-damaged sea lions got counted more accurately than us human beings. According to a 2010 *New York Post* article, "Christine Ren-Fielding, MD, admitted in an academic article that, because some patients die months afterward, 'the incidence of bariatric deaths in New York City is practically unknowable for us.' "[47] It's amazing to this li'l old fat lady that someone would actually make this statement when it's possible to do a nationwide tire recall.

The same *New York Post* article says the state is investigating NYU Medical Center's booming weight-loss surgery practice after three young patients perished. Ages for two of the three patients were listed as 25 and 27. The NYU Program for Surgical Weight Loss operates on almost 1,000 annually. "Bariatric procedures—which are advertised in city subways and take as little as 20 minutes to perform—are big moneymakers. NYU billed Rebecca Quatinetz [the 27-year-old who died] more than $26,000. Surgeons say their cut is often around $4,000."[48] So, with 1,000 surgeries, NYU Medical Center makes about $26 million annually, and the surgeons' cut is $4 million. Yes, bariatric surgery *is* a big moneymaker. Just take a look at what has happened since 1995.

Bariatric surgeries have exploded
in popularity.
The numbers nationally:

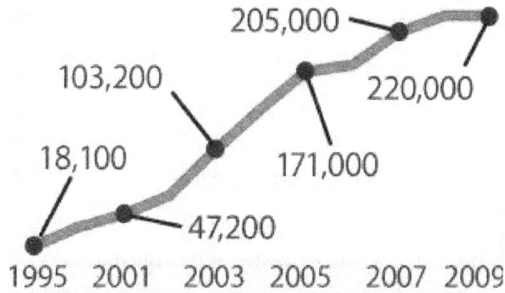

205,000

103,200

18,100

220,000

171,000

47,200

1995 2001   2003 2005   2007 2009

Sources: American Society for Metabolic &
Bariatric Surgery; University of Minnesota [49]

Now, let's do a little simple math here. Add up the surgeries from 1995 to 2009 and the number is 764,500. Multiply this number by NIDDK's latest *conservative* death rate estimate of 0.3% and you get 2,294 deaths from bariatric surgery from 1995 to 2009. Add in another guesstimated half million surgeries since 2009 and you get 1,264,500 surgeries and 3,794 deaths. Remember, that's a conservative number—the actual death toll from bariatric surgery is most likely higher. But no one is counting. And, unless you happen to be a family member or loved one of the victims who died, it's just a number.

Why in the world would desperate extremely obese folks choose this risky option? Because we Americans have been programmed to trust our medical professionals. Because it doesn't involve fundamental change. You just go in, sign the surgery liability release papers, and they wheel you off. *If* everything goes perfectly, you just keep eating the same foods that got you into trouble in the first place—but less of them. This resistance to fundamental change is a huge financial windfall for the bariatric surgeons, the hospitals, and the health care industry as a whole.

Contrast this to the "fundamental-change-hysterical-fear" routine that occurred back in 1973 when Dr. Robert C. Atkins dared to say that carbohydrates make us fat. Because a dietary change that says eat fewer carbohydrates and more proteins and fats (cholesterol) is fundamental, the result is the "Galileo Effect." We fear and attack fundamental change—it's just the way we humans are.

In comparison to the three young adults who died from bariatric surgery at the NYU Medical Center, let's take a look at this li'l old fat lady who didn't go down the bariatric surgery path. In contrast to the risks of dying, osteoporosis, and significant weight regain, I would have to say that my personal experience of losing weight slowly has been nothing less than spectacular. By defying current diet doctrine and eating a diet low in carbohydrates but high in essential proteins and essential fats, I was able to send diabetes and heart disease scurrying in retreat.

But folks can't see that—they can just see my appearance. So, let's speak to my appearance. Even though I began losing weight at age 52, it was slowly enough so that my body was able to adjust and I don't have drooping this and sagging that. People who haven't seen me for a while are sometimes speechless. I have learned to understand that folks who aren't friendly toward me probably just don't recognize me. When people do figure out who I am, a typical statement usually goes something like this. "You just look *soooo* good!"

Let me give you an example. While some local folks are aware that I have lost weight, others don't have a clue. One day at the post office I ran into two men. One man knew I had lost weight while the other man had no idea. The one man greeted me with my name and the man who was with him did a triple take and then just about fainted. I had worked with that man on a project when I was a li'l old fat lady, and he couldn't believe that the woman he was looking at was me. He was horrified because he knew that I knew what was going on inside his head. It was all I could do to not roll on the floor and laugh. His reaction was testament to my incredible transformation from a li'l old fat lady into a healthy, vibrant, sexy gal. I may be 61 years old and have a few gray hairs and wrinkles but, unlike the three young NYU Medical Center bariatric surgery victims, I'm nowhere near dead yet.

Now, I know that the corn growers and everyone else who peddles PSS-rich foods or makes a nice living off of sick obese folks are reading this in horror. Not to worry. Early on, I claimed that I would offer some realistic solutions so that the obese ill consumer could have his cake and eat it too, and so that many American businesses could make a lot of money. I'm going to keep this promise, but it involves a little bit of change. And I know how difficult that is going to be for some folks so I'm going to offer a strategy that will give those of us who don't want to change the ability to just stay the way we are. After all, this is the United States of America, the land of the free.

CHAPTER 4

My Deal With The Devil

If it looks like a duck, walks like a duck, and quacks like a duck, it must be a duck.—Multiple Authors

I have two adult daughters. When my younger daughter was about a year old, she would be playing contentedly and then suddenly become rigid, turn bright red, and then emit a terrifying scream. I was horrified. This happened several times, so I made an emergency appointment with her pediatrician.

He examined her and told me that the poor little thing had somehow become "stopped up." Unlike adults, who understand what is happening, my baby's solution was to try and resist the pain. The doctor said her situation was not yet harmful, but we needed to get her "unstopped."

Part of his solution was for me to feed her spoonfuls of mineral oil. I immediately rushed down to the little on-site pharmacy and located the mineral oil. As I was standing there holding the bottle of clear mineral oil, I realized that most of the oil would never reach its intended destination. Even as a baby, my little girl was very strong. She was too young to understand that swallowing the mineral oil would help her feel better, so she was going to violently resist taking it. Most of the oil was going to end up on her, me, the furniture, the walls, and the floor. What a nightmare!

Now, I have this kaleidoscope brain that takes little bits and pieces of information and comes up with out-of-the-box solutions. In this emergency, my brain went into overdrive, and it immediately formulated a plan that just might work. I bought the mineral oil and then went directly to the grocery store. There, I bought red food coloring, cherry flavoring, and liquid sweetener. I wouldn't normally feed my baby junk, but I was desperate.

Small children occasionally get ear infections. The medication of choice was generally amoxicillin, an antibiotic. Instead of a pill, the medication was contained in pink sweet liquid, and my daughter absolutely loved the way it tasted. If I could get the mineral oil to look and taste even vaguely similar to the amoxicillin, maybe I could avoid a certain disaster.

I hurried home and put a tiny amount of each of the ingredients I had purchased into the mineral oil. When I shook it up, the stuff turned milky pink just like the amoxicillin! I tasted it and made a couple of minor adjustments. Then, I called to my daughter in the same way I called to give her the amoxicillin.

She came running over, saw the bottle of pink liquid in my hand, and unhesitatingly swallowed the large spoonful of mineral oil. Then she happily took off and started playing again. The remaining doses of mineral oil went down just as easily.

A few days later we went back to the pediatrician. He pronounced her well and then slyly asked me about the mineral oil. She didn't object to taking it? I told him she loved it and his jaw dropped. Because I felt so smug, I brought the remaining oil with me to show him what I had done. The pediatrician broke into a huge grin and he told me that he would recommend my solution to all of his future patients with the same problem.

Even though my story is horribly tacky and tasteless, this experience taught me a valuable lesson. And it eventually helped *me* lose 90 pounds and become healthy. This is an example of the old saying, "If it looks like a duck, walks like a duck, and quacks like a duck, it must be a duck." If I am a fast food junkie and I eat low-PSS, "unleaded" foods that look and taste like the "leaded" fast food I love, I must be eating fast food. Right? It's the same principle.

Please don't ask carboholic Americans who eat a lot of fast food to "just do it" and start eating things like carrots and celery sticks. It's not going to happen. This kind of thinking flies in the face of Mother Nature. Carboholic fast food junkies will start eating foods that don't cause them to gain weight and get diseases when the food itself changes. It's the same for all those carboholic health nut folks who only eat organic but buy obscene quantities of carbohydrates at the health food stores.

This li'l old fat lady spent almost two decades honing her professional marketing skills at getting folks to adopt Discontinuous Innovations. So, I'm going to give you a cardinal rule I learned from the school-of-hard-knocks. The more you can make your Discontinuous Innovation look, taste, smell, feel, sound, and act like what folks are already accustomed to, the better. Here's an example of what *not* to do. A few years ago, Burger King tried to offer its customers a low-carb burger wrapped in a lettuce leaf. A burger is meat, cheese, and condiments that are placed between the top and bottom halves of a bun. A bun! Without the bun, there is no burger. Period. Even today, this li'l old fat lady cannot find a low-carb burger bun in the fast food joints. Nope, today all they're peddling is the "leaded" stuff.

Remember when my doctor diagnosed me with reactive hypoglycemia and gave me that single sheet of paper that had an "OK" food list and a "no-no" food list? Well, early on I struggled because there were so many familiar foods on the "no-no" list. Things like bread, sweets, cake, candy, ice cream, and chocolate. Things that I loved and had eaten all my life but that contained too much PSS. It was not a good time. I wanted to see, taste, and smell the same foods that I had grown up with. I was dealing with a brain that was addicted to all carbohydrates including the taste of sweet.

So, I became obsessed with finding low-PSS, "unleaded" alternatives for as many "no-no" foods as possible. I didn't need to pay any attention to calories and fat, so it became a wonderful bargain hunt. I was looking for PSS bargains. Now, my friends will tell you that I am a world class bargain hunter. One of my friends even refers to me as a Market Maven. This is a term used in Malcolm Gladwell's excellent book *The Tipping Point*, which looks at why major changes in our society so often happen suddenly and unexpectedly.[1] So, why not take my love of bargain hunting and leverage it into finding foods that allow me to have my cake and eat it too?

Let's pause here for a moment and think about the word "diet." When we think about losing weight, we think about dieting. Do you realize that the first three letters of the word "diet" spell *die*? Well, that's what could happen if we tried to stay on a real diet forever. So, we restrict our calorie and fat intake for a little while, lose the weight, and then go back to the same foods that got us into trouble in the first place. To repeat Einstein, *"The definition of insanity is doing the same thing over and over again and expecting different results."*

But, if we change the rules, we can have our cake and eat it too. Literally. We don't need to diet to lose weight and become healthy. We just need to change the rules from calorie and fat counting to carb counting. It's a bargain—you get two for the price of one. Or, another way of saying it is that you give up PSS, but you get calories and fat back. But wait! My bargain-hunting math is completely wrong. You actually get four back for the price of one. You get calories, fat, personal freedom, and health. And once you've learned what foods constitute carb bargains, you don't even need to count carbs. At least I don't—not anymore. I just eat what I want to eat, but it's almost always a carb bargain.

This sounds pretty simple. So, what's the rub? Well, it's sort of like trying to find "un-leaded" gasoline before 1975. Right now it's almost impossible to find PSS bargains on the grocery store shelves. I'm not exaggerating. Whole grocery store aisles are off limits.

Yes, we think we tried low carb in 2003. But, no, we didn't really do what I am recommending. Yes, what happened in 2003 was a feeble attempt at low carb, but it was also low calorie and low fat, too. It was just another temporary diet! And because it was low calorie and low fat, we consumers hated it. The low carb stuff sat on the shelves and rotted because we wouldn't buy it. We were still buying the "leaded" stuff that causes our pancreas to poison us.

Here's an example of one company that tried to introduce a low carb version of milk. A milk company named Hood introduced a product line called Carb Countdown. Hood offered it in 2%, fat free, and chocolate. I loved the stuff because it tasted like high-PSS milk but, instead of the 2% containing 12 grams of carbs per eight-ounce glass, it only contained three grams of carbs. A PSS bargain! Well, one day I noticed that Hood had changed the name of the product line. The carton looked the same but it was now called Calorie Countdown, not Carb Countdown. Why? Because we consumers wouldn't buy the low carb version, but we will buy *anything* that says "low calorie"! It's also more expensive than a comparable container of "leaded" milk, and that's a deterrent, too. I keep expecting my local grocery store to discontinue it because it's located down at the bottom of the cooler and they sell so little of it that the Use By dates are always expiring on the containers.

You may ask why we even need a low carb version of something natural like milk. Well, almost all of the milk we drink comes from specially bred high production milk cows. And then we strip the fat out of it so that the 12 grams of sugar takes a short cut to our pancreas. When we're trying to fix our weight problem, or if you are hypersensitive to PSS like me, there's just too much sugar in cow's milk. Natural cheese that's produced from cow's milk doesn't contain hardly any sugar, but it contains lots of fat and calories, so many Americans avoid real cheese like the plague. So why do I even want to drink milk if it's got too much sugar? Because I grew up drinking milk and I love it on my low PSS, "unleaded" cereal. I want to have my cake and eat it too.

The same goes for heavy whipped cream. Land-O-Lakes makes a rich, high fat, high calorie, low PSS version. But we consumers wouldn't buy this wonderful product either. It just sat on the shelves and rotted while we consumers bought the "leaded" version to top our pies and other sweets. For a while, four of the Super Walmarts in the Denver area of Colorado stocked the item. They finally gave up, and Land-O-Lakes tells me they don't show a single retailer in the entire state of Colorado offering the product.[2] Now, the only grocery retailer that will special order it for me is Walmart. I get it by taking an empty container to a nearby Walmart so they can scan the UPC (bar code) to see if the number is still in their computer database. If the number is there, Walmart will special order it in for me so I can get my Land-O-Lakes whipped cream by the 12-can case. Yes, I buy 12 cans at a time. Fortunately, it has a very long shelf life, so Walmart gets a gold star for this one.

Many of the items I use to keep my PSS intake down are currently only available online. And, because they are "specialty items," they are generally more expensive than their high PSS "leaded" counterparts that most Americans are putting into their grocery carts. It would be really nice if I could just write up my little grocery list, hop in the car, and run down the nearest grocery store. But I can't. That's the price I pay for defying current diet doctrine.

So, what's my Deal With The Devil? Like with the mineral oil, I've struck a deal with the devil regarding carbohydrate-rich comfort foods and stuff that is sweet. I grew up eating obscene amounts of carbohydrates and rich sweets and still crave them, even after eight years of eating a low PSS diet. So, I've learned to substitute low PSS "unleaded" versions of comfort foods and to sweeten my rich calorie laden desserts with low PSS "unleaded" sweeteners that my taste buds tell me is sweet. I have my cake and eat it too. Here is a Peggy Prediction repeat.

Peggy Prediction: *Based upon my own weight loss journey, I found it very easy to break the physical metabolic addiction to excessive sweets and carbohydrates. But, like alcoholism, nicotine, and other addictions, fixing the disturbances in my brain's reward circuits proved very difficult. So I predict that, after consuming excessive carbohydrates for many decades, the brain's abnormal, addicted desire for carbohydrates and the taste of sweet is almost impossible to break. That's why I have my cake and eat it too.*

Now, I realize that many Americans think that the low PSS "unleaded" versions of sweets are artificial. We even call the low PSS versions "artificial" sweeteners. But, many of them are now made from natural things like corn. Yes, corn. Hello, Corn Refiners Association! Are you listening? All you need to do is get smarter about getting the PSS out of your corn. You can turn your corn from being a low-price commodity into a high-price commodity by making more profitable low PSS "unleaded" products. You can make more money! You think I'm joking? I'm not. If you will help consumers become normal weight and healthy, they will pay you handsomely. It's sort of the Starbucks pricing model for corn. C'mon now. You need to start thinking outside the box. This is true for you wheat farmers, too. Later on in this chapter, I'll tell you about a wonderful wheat-based product that is also a low PSS.

Unfortunately, many of the companies that are working to develop these low PSS "unleaded" versions of sweeteners have scientists and engineers in charge. So they are focused on making a wonderful product, but not on how to get the consumer to actually buy it. A simple thing like a warm, fuzzy, natural-sounding name would make a big difference. I know it shouldn't, but that is how we consumers are. They haven't developed good retail distribution channels, either. If the product name sounds like a chemical and folks can't buy it easily, most customers will go elsewhere.

Even though many Americans prefer "natural leaded" sugar over low PSS "artificial unleaded" sweeteners, I'll let you in on a dirty little secret. "Natural" sugar is far from natural. Do you have any idea what "natural" sugar goes through before you dump copious quantities into your ice tea? It's horrifying. For one thing, table sugar made from both sugar cane and beets is produced using lime. Yes, that alkaline substance that makes the rings around your toilet. The little brown "natural" sugar packets aren't really any better. They just make some folks feel better about their carboholism.

What about Splenda? (Now, *that's* a warm, fuzzy, natural-sounding name!) Don't lots of Americans use that widely available low PSS sweetener? Yes, we do, and it's wonderful to have that relatively low PSS sweetener available. But wait! While it's a low PSS compared to regular sugar, most folks don't realize that Johnson & Johnson has bulked up its product to resemble regular table sugar by adding not one, but two sugars in sheep's clothing. They're called dextrose and maltodextrin. So, a cup of Splenda actually contains 24 grams of carbs.[3] The sucralose in the Splenda contains zero grams of carbs, but Johnson & Johnson is a smart marketing company, so they bulk up their product to resemble table sugar. (To be completely accurate, the little packets of Splenda contain dextrose, maltodextrin, and sucralose in that order, which means that more than two-thirds of the ingredients by volume are sugars. The big bags contain maltodextrin and sucralose, in that order.)

By bulking the sucralose up with low-cost sugars, Johnson & Johnson makes consumers think we're getting more low PSS product for our money and we also don't have to change our habits. We just measure out the Splenda in the same quantities as table sugar. How simple is that? But we've just put 24 grams of unnecessary PSS per cup of Splenda into our foods and eventually into our stomachs. Could Johnson & Johnson not put the added sugar into their product? Yes, but that wouldn't maximize their profits.

As a smart marketing company, you always worry about "cannibalization" of your product lines. That means you don't introduce one product at the expense of another, even if it's in the best interests of your customer. According to www.about.com, "Since the manufacturer of Splenda has held back on making a liquid [low PSS] form available (despite numerous letter-writing campaigns and petitions), a cottage industry has grown to provide sucralose in liquid forms."[4] Now, while I've had a little fun with Johnson & Johnson, please let me emphasize this point. Johnson & Johnson is a smart, successful company. They're successful because they deliver products that we consumers will buy. If we want Johnson & Johnson to change their products, that change needs to be driven by you and me. We're the consumers, and we're in charge.

So, if you want sucralose that doesn't contain sugar in sheep's clothing, you have to go online to buy it. By volume, sucralose is 600 times as sweet as table sugar. One drop equals one packet of Splenda. The equivalent of one cup of sugar is 24 drops. Various trade names include Sweetzfree, EZ-Sweetz, Fiberfit, and Liquid Sucralose by Healthy Cheat Foods. There is lots of information on these sweeteners at www.about.com. Speaking of www.about.com, this website contains all sorts of useful information that will help you take control of your weight and health. The website is www.lowcarbdiets.about.com.

A relative newcomer that has entered the sweetener fray is Stevia in the Raw, made by Cumberland Packing Corporation. Cumberland also makes Sugar in the Raw and Agave in the Raw, which appeals to those organic-type consumers. Unfortunately, the majority ingredients in this product are dextrose in the packets and maltodextrin in the "baker's bag," both sugars in sheep's clothing. Unfortunately, when I looked at the Nutrition Facts tab on the manufacturer's website, I couldn't find any product ingredients listed.[5] I had to look at the actual product in the store to know what's in Stevia in the Raw. So, it looks like Cumberland is trying to jump on Splenda's bandwagon of bulking up their product with low-cost sugar. On the other hand, Cargill, with its Truvia (erythritol and stevia) product, is truly offering consumers a low PSS product. There's no sugar in sheep's clothing listed on their nutrition label.[6]

One observation I've made of my carboholic friends is that many of them keep saying they don't like the taste of low PSS "unleaded" sweeteners. Now maybe I've eaten so much of the stuff for so long that my taste buds have learned to translate. So, I decided to do a little primary marketing research to see if people could actually taste the difference. The Safeway Select Watch'n Carbs product is a full-fat premium ice cream that is sweetened with Splenda, and it tastes wonderful to me.

I went out and bought a container of the Safeway Select Watch'n Carbs Vanilla Bean along with a container of Breyers Natural Vanilla, Kroger Private Selection Crushed Vanilla Bean, Open Nature 100% Natural Vanilla Bean, and Safeway Select Vanilla Bean. I put one-quarter-cup samples of these five ice creams into little cups with color-coded dots and had 15 people taste them to see if they could pick out the ice cream that was sweetened with Splenda. I told my research group that their task was to pick out the one ice cream that was sweetened with Splenda instead of sugar.

Now, if there was no difference in taste, the odds dictate that three of the 15 people would pick out the Splenda-sweetened ice cream. I know my sample size was too small to be statistically significant, but if a large percentage of my 15 taste testers picked out the Splenda-sweetened ice cream, it would still indicate to me that there was indeed some difference in taste. Here are my results. Only two tasters picked out the Safeway Select Watch'n Carbs Vanilla Bean ice cream that is sweetened with Splenda.

Interestingly, six tasters picked the Open Nature 100% Natural Vanilla Bean that is sweetened with sugar. My hypothesis is that the Open Nature 100% Natural ice cream doesn't taste as good as the other four ice creams, so my taste testers picked it out because they think that low PSS ice cream won't taste as good as the "leaded" stuff.

Based on the ice cream taste test results, I believe that rich, good-tasting sweets can be made with those nasty "unleaded" sweeteners. If anyone wants to challenge my results with a big expensive scientific research project, please be my guest.

I've also heard many people say that they can definitely taste the difference between diet soda and regular soda. I suspect that they are right. Why? Because the biggies, Coke and Pepsi, sweeten their diet sodas with aspartame. Aspartame is made from *methyl ester of the aspartic acid/phenylalanine dipeptide.* Now, try and repeat that name three times. I bet you can't.

This li'l old fat lady believes that many folks would find the low PSS "unleaded" versions of soda much more acceptable if Coke and Pepsi used one of the newer sweeteners that are made from natural things like corn. They're already making their "leaded" soda with corn-based fructose. So, why don't Coke and Pepsi make their diet sodas with the newer "unleaded" corn-based sweeteners? It's all about money. Aspartame currently costs a lot less than the newer sweeteners. And, like Johnson & Johnson, Coke and Pepsi don't want to cannibalize their cheap "leaded" fructose-sweetened products. Just imagine what would happen to their corporate profits if they used more expensive "unleaded" sweeteners that made their low PSS "unleaded" sodas just as good as their cheap "leaded" sodas. Not only would their production costs increase for the diet soda, but less people would be buying the regular soda. It's a double financial whammy. Nope, Coke and Pepsi will keep using *methyl ester of the aspartic acid/phenylalanine dipeptide* until it's no longer economically beneficial for them.

Now, you may be questioning why I keep using the terms "leaded" and "unleaded" in this chapter. Here's why. Tetraethyllead, abbreviated TEL, is a lead *added* to gasoline that is readily absorbed into the skin on contact or into the lungs from automotive exhaust. Lead pollution from engine exhaust is dispersed into the air and into the vicinity of roads and is easily inhaled. Lead is a toxic metal that accumulates and, especially at low exposure levels, has subtle and insidious neurotoxic effects, such as low IQ and antisocial behavior. It has particularly harmful effects on children.[7] Here's a little bit of American history written by William Kovarik, professor at Radford University in Virginia.

> GM started marketing its "Ethyl" (leaded gasoline) fluid in 1923. In 1924 it joined with Standard Oil (Exxon) to form a partnership called the Ethyl Corp. Since DuPont was a one-third owner of GM at the time, the three major corporations all had a hand in the development and marketing of leaded gasoline. Other companies quickly joined in, including Andrew Mellon's Gulf Oil Co. with an exclusive contract for Southeastern US distribution of leaded gasoline. Mellon was Secretary of Treasury during this time and in charge of the Public Health Service, which was investigating leaded gasoline.

> The public controversy started when about five workers at a grossly unsafe Standard Oil refinery went violently insane in 1924. Many others

were also hospitalized. Public health experts, including Alice Hamilton of Harvard and Yendell Henderson of Yale, vehemently opposed the use of lead in gasoline as a menace to public health. Henderson called it "the single most important question in the field of public health that has ever faced the American public."

In 1925 the Public Health Service convened a conference on leaded gasoline. The structure of the conference was slanted towards industry, which may have had something to do with the influence of Andrew Mellon. At the conference, Hamilton called GM vice-president Charles Kettering "nothing but a murderer" for distributing leaded gasoline. Lead poisoning, as Hamilton knew, had been a familiar and dreaded "occupational disease" throughout centuries of European history. Hamilton also insisted that there were other ways to get an anti-knock (higher octane) fuel.

Kettering and others, speaking for GM and Standard Oil (which together had created the Ethyl Corp. early in 1924) claimed that they did not know of alternatives "in the paraffin series" that gave anti-knock results. Frank Howard of Standard went much further, saying that civilization rested on engines and fuels, and that (in his immortal words) leaded gasoline had come "like a gift from heaven."

Starting in 1975 and concluding in 1986, leaded gasoline was phased out by government order in the United States. It was also banned in various European nations in the 1990s. It is still having serious public health impacts in developing nations, and a complete global phase-out has long been advocated by the World Health Organization and all other international health organizations.

…Leaded gasoline should be counted among the great environmental disasters of the 20th century, given the numbers of people killed or slowly poisoned by the dull grey metal. Significantly, alternatives were well known from the beginning and preferred by the same researchers who created leaded gasoline. They originally saw it as nothing more than a bridge to other, safer fuels. Leaded gasoline was phased out in the US from 1975-1986 and in Europe in the 1990s. It is still being used in the developing world.[8]

So, for 50 years (1925–1975), our leaders in Washington caved to big business regarding knowingly putting poisonous lead into our gasoline. And history always repeats itself. Here's the current version of poisonous lead, but this time it's in our food in the form of excessive carbohydrates. In 1973, Dr. Robert C. Atkins stood up in front of the US Senate Select Committee and testified that carbohydrates make us fat. He was vilified and labeled a fraud. That was over 39 years ago. Unfortunately, much of what Atkins predicted has turned out to be completely true. (The official record of this event can be obtained at www.hathitrust.org by searching under "nutrition and diseases 1973.") More than 200 million Americans are now overweight or obese, and the rates of diabetes, heart disease, hypertension, and more continue to skyrocket. With so many Americans sick and dying from the effects of excessive carbohydrate consumption, the cost of health care in America has become completely obscene, with Kaiser projecting the 2011 annual insurance premium cost for family coverage to be $15,520 (200-plus workers).[9]

Let me take the liberty of modifying Kovarik's last statement just a little. *"Leaded" foods should be counted among the great dietary disasters of the 20th and 21st centuries, given the numbers of people killed or slowly poisoned by the* real *bad boy on the block.* And let me take the liberty of quoting Yendell Henderson of Yale who vehemently opposed the use of lead in gasoline in 1925 as a menace to public health. Henderson called it *"the single most important question in the field of public health that has ever faced the American public."* History always repeats itself.

The only real difference between 1925 and 2012 is, rather than adding a poison to our gasoline, we have added excessive carbohydrates to almost all of our foods, which makes our magnificent pancreas slowly poison us to death. What makes this situation all the more tragic is that our processed food industries tried to get on the low carbohydrate bandwagon that occurred during 2003. Big business would have continued to expand our low PSS "unleaded" food options if consumers had rewarded them by purchasing the stuff. But the large majority of consumers would have none of it. I personally watched one "low carb" product after another disappear from the grocery store shelves because consumers wouldn't purchase it.

So, if you are fed up with being obese and sick, you are the one who must take responsibility for yourself. You are the one who must defy current diet doctrine to regain your health and personal freedom. Please don't expect our government or big business to put your personal interests first. Their top priorities are to do things that will fuel the American economy and maximize next quarter's earnings. Don't expect either of them to do something that might contradict this reality.

While this may sound harsh, it's this American economic system that has made our country a powerhouse in the world for so many decades. If we want to turn the tide of obesity and ill health, it's up to each of us consumers to make this happen. Later, this li'l old fat lady will offer up some solutions that would allow obese ill consumers to have their cake and eat it too, while enabling many big businesses to generate nice profits for their stockholders.

But, back to "leaded" foods. As a very PSS sensitive person, I have discovered that excessive carbs lurk in almost all of our processed foods. Sometimes in obscene quantities. For example, take Honey Nut Cheerios, which are made by General Mills. The TV ads for Honey Nut Cheerios trumpet that their wonderful oat cereal is good for your heart. Small quantities of unprocessed oats probably do benefit the heart in some way. But they've added so much sugar that there's 20 grams of carbohydrate in a single three-quarter-cup serving of Honey Nut Cheerios![10] Don't forget to add another 12 grams of carbohydrates for a cup of milk. Do the math. One single serving of cereal with a cup of milk contains 32 grams of carbs! My arteries feel like they are starting to clog just thinking about it.

I had to do some soul searching to figure out why this particular Honey Nut Cheerios TV ad was so offensive to me. I think it's because General Mills represents that Honey Nut Cheerios are good for your heart. Anything that contains 32 grams of carbs in a single serving will contribute to obesity, diabetes, hypertension, and heart disease. So, according to my nose, the TV ad just doesn't pass the smell test.

Now, in defense of the Honey Nut Cheerios product, it's definitely not the worst of its kind. The Kellogg's Mini-Wheats Bite Size cereal with advertising that's targeted toward our precious little children comes with your choice of white, blue, or pink sugar frosting. A single 25-biscuit serving of this cereal contains approximately 41 grams of carbs.[11] Add 12 grams of carbs for the milk, and your little child has just ingested 53 grams of carbs. And that's before the large glass of orange juice. The "natural" healthy hot cereals have similar carb counts.

Peggy Prediction: *I'm betting that when America's parents finally stop feeding their precious little children obscene amounts of PSS, ADHD may lose some of its popularity.*

Another gimmick is the phrase "Sugar Free." Don't allow yourself to be fooled. Sugar free doesn't mean carb free. This is one of the reasons I've adopted the term "PSS." The *real* bad boy on the block can't hide if you use PSS.

Here's an example. Because I can only get my favorite ice cream in two flavors (vanilla and butter pecan), I add things like low PSS cookies, nuts, and candy to the vanilla flavor. At the grocery store one day, I spotted jars of Smucker's caramel ice cream topping that blared "Sugar Free" in big letters on the front label. My heart did a little skip because I thought maybe I had discovered another carb bargain. The ugly truth was on the nutrition label. The first ingredient was maltodextrin (a sugar in sheep's clothing), so two tablespoons of this "Sugar Free" ice cream topping had 11 grams of carbs.[12] I know I'm a pig, but I don't drizzle two tablespoons of topping on my ice cream. By the time I got done drizzling four tablespoons of topping on my low carb ice cream, my dessert would contain 25 grams of carbs. No thank you.

But, maybe I'm just an ungrateful wretch. Maybe I should be *happy* with 25 grams of carbs. Why? Because, compared to the *regular* Smucker's caramel ice cream topping, maybe Smucker's considers it to be sugar free. Let me lay out the obesity, diabetes, hypertension, and heart disease facts. Two tablespoons of the regular Smucker's caramel ice cream topping contains 30 grams of carbs.[13] So, four tablespoons of topping along with one-half cup of regular vanilla ice cream would set me back about 75 grams of carbs. I don't usually consume that many carbs in two days. So, let's see here, one little dessert or two full days of eating lots of wonderful, rich, high calorie, high fat foods. Nope, I think I'll just stick with my strategy to have my cake and eat it too.

OK, so I use low PSS sweeteners to keep my carb counts low. But what about all the other stuff in the rich baked goods I eat? Like the flour. Doesn't it have lots of carbs, too? Absolutely. But, there's a company out there called Tova Industries that makes this wonderful product called Carbquik.[14] Unlike Bisquick, which contains 75 grams net carbs per cup, Tova Industries states that their Carbquik product contains six net carbs per cup. It's so unbelievable that I even contacted Tova Industries to verify their carb number. Tova Industries confirmed that they had used an independent testing company to calculate the nutritional values of Carbquik and they would stand behind their number.[15]

Now, I think this may be a good time to explain some of the intricacies of the nutrition labels on the back of all of our processed foods. The word "Carbohydrates" usually gets broken down further into words like "Sugar," "Fiber," "Sugar Alcohols," etc. *The way to get to the PSS (net carb) count is to take carbohydrates and subtract out fiber and sugar alcohols. All of the other carb stuff will cause our pancreas to produce insulin.*

Using Carbquik and Bisquick as examples, a cup of Carbquik (96 grams) has 48 grams of carbs, of which 42 grams are fiber.[16] That means a net carb count of six grams per cup. A cup of Bisquick (120 grams) has a carb count of 78 grams, of which three grams are fiber.[17] That means a net carb count of 75 grams per cup. So, we've got 75 grams of net carbs versus six grams of net carbs. Carbquik is a carb bargain. For me, the Carbquik is truly a miracle product because it produces baked goods that taste pretty much the same as the "leaded" stuff.

But it doesn't always produce baked goods exactly like regular flour, and I sometimes take my whole experimental batch of something and throw it out. It also has a manufacturers' suggested retail price (MSRP) of $18.95 for a three-pound box and must be ordered online. A six-pound box of Bisquick can be purchased from Costco for $5.49. I've managed to find Carbquik online at netrition.com for $11.99 plus shipping. That would make the price without shipping $4.00/per pound for the Carbquik and $.92/pound for the Bisquick. So, the Carbquik costs over four times as much per pound. But, it allows me to have my cake and eat it too, so I go online and order at least three boxes of Carbquik at a time along with other low PSS essentials that are not available at my local grocery store. Wheat farmers! Are you listening? Just look at the price I'm paying for your commodity!

So, we've got a low PSS count for the sweetener and the flour in baked goods. That just leaves the remaining recipe ingredients. With a little diligence, it is possible to make wonderful foods and desserts that will knock your socks off without making your pancreas become toxic.

One issue I haven't yet addressed is the fear that the "unleaded" sweeteners I use might possibly be toxic. This unsubstantiated fear is a perfect example of the "fundamental-change-hysterical-fear" routine. It's becoming harder to remember but, a few decades ago, there was all sorts of hysteria that we would perish from using microwave ovens. Today, there are very few households that don't have a microwave oven. For eight years I have been using low PSS sweeteners. For eight years I have looked in vain for the warning labels associated with using these foods.

But the warning labels associated with my Lipitor go on and on. If you actually *listen* to the drug ads on TV, most of the air time is spent telling you how much damage they can do to your body. As a matter of fact, I am now sporting an artificial lens in my right eye because of taking prescribed steroids for pain caused by a congenital issue (birth defect) with some vertebra in my neck. At least that is what the ophthalmic surgeon told me. Two years earlier, my eye exam didn't indicate a hint of cataracts. The adverse reaction of "Posterior Subcapsular Cataracts" was number 38 on a list of 41 potential hazards itemized on that little paper that comes with all of our prescriptions. You should try *reading* that little paper word for word sometime. It's a real eye opener. Surgery fixed the congenital vertebra issue and the new "turbocharged" multifocal artificial lens in my right eye has completely freed me up from wearing eye glasses, so I really don't have anything to complain about. But I have become much more wary of taking any prescription medications or over-the-counter drugs.

So, back to those nasty "unleaded" sweeteners that might possibly be toxic. Based upon my eight years of personal experience as a human guinea pig who has lost 90 pounds, avoided becoming diabetic, and no longer needs to take prescription Lipitor or other medications to control my high cholesterol and avoid heart disease, I'll take this "risk." I also feel great joy every day because I eat what I want when I want and have regained my personal freedom and health. So, I'm very happy with my Deal With The Devil.

 Now, this seems like a good time to list some of our common carbohydrates and sweeteners by name and type. So, I'm going to give you the li'l old fat lady version and try to not make your eyes cross too much.

When dealing with PSS stuff, we need to know that carbohydrates come in three flavors. The three big names are monosaccharides, disaccharides, and polysaccharides. "Mono" means one, "di" means two, and "poly" means three or more.

All this means is that the "mono" versions are something that your body absorbs directly into your bloodstream during digestion. They are the simplest form of sugar (carbohydrate). Examples of monosaccharides include glucose (dextrose), fructose (levulose), galactose, xylose, and ribose.

Monosaccharides are the building blocks of disaccharides, such as sucrose, lactose, and maltose. For example, sucrose (table sugar) is made up of glucose and fructose. Lactose (milk sugar) is made up of glucose and galactose. Maltose (grain sugar) is made up of two units of glucose. Your body has to do a tiny bit more work to get them into your bloodstream.

Then, there are the polysaccharides, which are sometimes called complex sugars. These include starch (such as corn, wheat, potatoes, and rice) and cellulose (such as fiber). These require your body to do even a little more work to get them into your bloodstream, and the fiber just doesn't get into your bloodstream at all (which is really, really good).

Now, when I say a little more work, that's exactly what I mean. *With the exception of fiber, the "-rides" all take your pancreas for a wild ride.*

So, why am I spouting all of these 15-letter words? Because you need to have a clue about all of these carbohydrates and sweeteners that are being loaded into our foods. This is the vocabulary on the back label of all that processed food you are buying. And then eating!

As I mentioned earlier, "sugar free" does not necessarily mean "carb free." So I'm going to rip off the sheep's clothing so you can see the naked animal. These are the sometimes weird-looking names that you will see on the nutrition label. Because they all are high PSS and stimulate your pancreas to produce insulin, they are all obesity-, diabetes-, high-blood-pressure-, and heart-disease-producing ingredients when they are consumed in large quantities for decades.

If you actually read the little nutrition label that's on just about everything you put in your shopping cart, you will be hard pressed to not see these words. Why do food processors put these gobbledygook names in our foods? Because they are extremely cheap and we Americans have developed a taste for them. Remember, we're the consumers and we're in charge.

Partial List of PSS in Sheep's Clothing

Agave syrup	Dextrin	Glucose	Maltose	Starch
Brown rice syrup	Dextrose	High-fructose corn syrup	Mannose	Sucrose
Cane juice	Dulcitol	Honey	Maple syrup	Syrup
Carob	Evaporated cane juice	Lactose	Molasses	Treacle
Corn sweeteners	Fructose	Levulose	Saccharose	Turbinado
Corn syrup	Fruit juice concentrate	Maltodextrin	Sorghum	Xylose

Interestingly, *Dr. Bernstein's Diabetes Solution* book says that "sugar alcohols" such as erythritol, maltitol, mannitol, sorbitol, and xylitol will raise a diabetic's blood sugars significantly when consumed by the tablespoon.[18] But, *The Art and Science of Low Carbohydrate Living*, by Jeff S. Volek, PhD, RD, and Stephen D. Phinney, MD, PhD, states that xylitol will not raise your insulin level.[19] So, even the experts in this field don't always completely agree. Since this li'l old fat lady has successfully used several of these sugar alcohols during my 90-pound weight loss journey, I'm not going to call them PSS in Sheep's Clothing. But, if you're a diabetic, I suggest you follow Dr. Bernstein's recommendation to check your blood sugars.

Here is a chart of our most common sweeteners, along with their technical name, PSS impact, what they're generally made from, some current trade names, and negative long-term side effects from eating lots and lots of them for decades. Much of the information is gleaned from Wikipedia. Just realize that this chart will continue to morph and grow as newer and better low PSS sweeteners become available.

Technical Name	PSS Impact	Commonly Produced From	Trade Names	Possible Negative Side Effects if Consumed in *Very Large* Quantities
Sucrose	High	Sugar cane, sugar beets	Sugar	Health problems including obesity, insulin resistance (diabetes), high blood pressure, coronary heart disease, and tooth decay.
Fructose	High	Sugar cane, sugar beets, corn	Sugar	Health problems including obesity, insulin resistance (diabetes), high blood pressure, coronary heart disease, and tooth decay. Digestive problems, including excessive flatulence, loose stools, and diarrhea.

Saccharine	Low	Benzoic sulfilimine	Sweet'N Low	In a December 14, 2010, release, the EPA stated that saccharin is no longer considered a potential hazard to human health.
Aspartame	Low	Methyl ester of the aspartic acid/phe-nylalanine dipeptide	NutraSweet, AminoSweet	A 2007 medical review on the subject concluded that "the weight of the existing scientific evidence indicates that aspartame is safe at current levels of consumption as a nonnutritive sweetener." It should be avoided by people with PKU.
Neotame	Low	Similar to Aspartame	Made by NutraSweet	Approved by FDA in July 2002. Sweeter than Aspartame, so less required
Sucralose	Low	Sucrose	Splenda, Sukrana, SucraPlus, Candys, Cukren, Nevella, Sweetzfree, EZ-Sweetz, Fiberfit, and Liquid Sucralose by Healthy Cheat Foods	No negative side effects listed. But, watch out for the PSS in sheep's clothing that's often added to the powdered sucralose.

Stevia	Low	*Stevia rabaudiana* plant		Used in Japan beginning in 1970. Beginning in 2009, the FDA considers it to be Generally Recognized as Safe. No negative side effects listed.
Erythritol	Low	Glucose	Zerose	In general, erythritol is free of side effects in regular use, but, if consumed in very large quantities, can have a laxative effect.
Stevia and Erythritol	Low	Glucose and *Stevia rabaudiana* plant	Truvia, PureVia	See stevia and erythritol.
Sorbitol	Low	Glucose	Sorbidex	Bloating, flatulence, and diarrhea. May aggravate irritable bowel syndrome, and similar gastrointestinal conditions.
Maltitol	Low	Maltose, corn	Maltidex	Bloating, flatulence, and diarrhea.
Mannitol	Low	Fructose	Mannidex	Bloating, flatulence, and diarrhea.
Isomalt	Low	Glucose and mannitol	Isomaltidex	Bloating, flatulence, and diarrhea.

Xylitol	Low	Cornhusk, cane pulp, seed hulls, cellulose of wood		Bloating, flatulence, and diarrhea. But is more easily tolerated than mannitol and sorbitol.
Tagatose	???	Milk, dairy products	Naturlose	Approved by FDA in October 2003. Dr. Bernstein unsure of PSS impact. [20]

So, what the heck does this chart and all its gobbledygook mean? It just means that our "leaded " natural sweeteners have a high PSS impact and cause significant health problems like obesity, diabetes, high blood pressure, heart disease, and more if we eat way too much of them for decades. Many of the older ones like saccharin and aspartame have chemical-sounding names, and many of the newer ones are generally made from natural things that we can pronounce.

Many of the newer "unleaded" natural ones are derived from the same sweeteners that cause our obesity and health problems. But the scientists have figured out how to make them a low or moderate PSS so we can have our cake and eat it too. The sucralose, stevia, and tagatose don't have any negative side effects listed. If we eat way too much of the remainder of them, we may not feel real good and have to go open the windows.

Right now, I'd have to say that Cargill is currently a leader in the marketing of "unleaded" natural sweeteners. They are the makers of Isomaltidex (isomalt), Maltidex (maltitol), Mannidex (mannitol), Sorbidex (sorbitol), Zeros (erythritol), and Truvia (stevia and erythritol). And Cargill is testing out Treha (trehalose) that might be "incorporated as part of a sports beverage system."[21] With the exception of Truvia, Cargill currently only wholesales its products to the food industry. But Cargill has clearly got some outside-the-box folks assigned to new product development, and I'd say that they're hedging their bets. My hat's off to you Cargill. May you beat the pants off your competition. Competition, put your pants on and go after Cargill.

For the past eight years, the "unleaded" natural sweeteners I have used the most are liquid sucralose and powdered erythritol. That doesn't mean that the others are not also good. Speaking of good, I understand the purist mind-set that our nutritional experts need to maintain. After all, they are nutrition professionals who must recommend only foods that provide "good" nourishment. But, like adding a tiny amount of food coloring, flavor, and sweetener to get my little girl to consume mineral oil that would help her get healthy, maybe it might make sense to consider embracing "unleaded" sweeteners that are made from natural things we can pronounce.

Is it possible that some of us low carb folks have the same mind-set on "unleaded" natural sweeteners that we are condemning in folks who can't see the forest for the trees regarding excess "leaded " natural carbohydrates in our foods? Because I'm just a li'l old fat lady, maybe I can get away with asking this question. My challenge to anyone who turns up his or her nose at the current generation of "unleaded" natural sweeteners is to produce the high-caliber scientific studies that link these low PSS sweeteners to the obesity epidemic with its diabetes, heart disease, high blood pressure, cancer, Alzheimer's disease, and more.

But why don't we just tell people to suck it up and eat healthy? Because that flies in the face of Mother Nature. If we want fast food junkies to change their eating habits, we need to change the food. All we need to do is get the high PSS content out of our processed foods and the fast food junkies will beat a path to our door.

However, the foods need to look and taste pretty much the same as what we're already accustomed to eating. This is the secret to implementing a fundamental change. Remember, "If it looks like a duck, walks like a duck, and quacks like a duck, it must be a duck." Another way of saying this is, "If it looks like a Big Mac and tastes like a Big Mac, then it must be a Big Mac." Burger King's burger wrapped in a lettuce leaf was an insult to all red-blooded fast food junkies. If it's called a burger, it's absolutely got to have a bun.

So, my secret to losing 90 pounds and regaining my health was, "If it looks like a duck, walks like a duck, and quacks like a duck, it must be a duck." By allowing myself to "have my cake and eat it too," I permanently changed what I ate without defying Mother Nature. Replacing high PSS foods with very similar low PSS foods enabled me to make my eating changes permanent without eliminating the foods I had grown up with and loved. At this point, there are only a few high PSS foods (french fries, for example) that I have given up. Because there are only a few, I've managed to turn my back on them because I value my personal freedom and health so much more. This li'l old fat lady even dreams that, one of these days, I'll be able to eat french fries again. In chapter 10, "Just One Fourth of a Penny," I'll offer a marketing strategy that could make this dream come true.

PART II

ADDITIONAL THINGS TO HELP YOU WIN YOUR HEALTH AND FREEDOM

CHAPTER 5

Exercise Should Be a Four-Letter Word

There are no data on weight loss when you go to a health club, either.
—Thomas Wadden, a University of Pennsylvania weight-loss expert[1]

I don't exercise. I never have and never will. I've finally accepted this fact, and it's made a huge improvement in my life.

I don't know about you, but in my younger years, I spent quite a bit of my hard-earned money on gym memberships and then failed to follow through. The ugly pattern was always the same. First, I got disgusted with my weight and physical condition. Then, I visited a nearby pay-for-use gym and was very impressed with the salesperson's tour of the magnificent machines that would make me thin and sleek. There always seemed to be some beautiful folks using these machines, and I envisioned myself looking just like them. If I exercised enough, I too would be thin and sleek. So, I would buy a membership, go faithfully to the gym for a short while, and then quit going.

The pay-for-use gyms depend on our failure for their success. Yes, that's right. The current gym business model would not work if each one of us who plunked down our hard-earned money actually went to the gym every day. There wouldn't be enough space and equipment to serve the hoards of people who showed up. So, the gyms sell lots of cheap memberships knowing that a significant percentage of the customers will not show up on a regular basis. The relatively few customers who actually do succeed in getting their backside down to the gym are getting a great bargain while the rest of us just spend our money. But don't blame the gyms. Remember, we're the consumers and we're in charge.

The grim Centers for Disease Control statistics on physical activity in this country state that only about 31% of Americans report they engage in regular leisure-time physical activity (defined as either three sessions per week of vigorous physical activity lasting 20 minutes or more, or five sessions per week of light-to-moderate physical activity lasting 30 minutes or more). About 40% of adults report no leisure-time physical activity. According to the National Institutes of Health, in contrast to reported activity, when physical activity is measured by a device that detects movement, only about 3–5% of adults obtain 30 minutes of moderate or greater intensity physical activity on at least five days per week.[2] Sounds to me like some folks are sandbagging when it comes to reporting leisure-time physical activity.

So, I would say that I used to be a pretty typical American. Having said this, at 61 years old, I am now much more physically active than I ever was in my younger years. How can I possibly be physically active if I say I don't exercise? Because I've found a couple of physical activities that, to me, are not physical exercise, but physical entertainment. Yes, there's a difference—a huge one for most of us.

The biggest difference between physical exercise and physical entertainment is the goal. The primary goal of physical exercise is the exercise. The primary goal of physical entertainment is the entertainment. This may sound like a shallow play on words, but the difference between the two is huge. Most of us exercise because it is good for us, not because it is incredibly pleasurable. Remember Mother Nature? Like eating things that are good for us rather than eating things that taste good? "Just do it" just doesn't work for most of us regarding eating *or* exercise.

Let me give you an example. I have a friend who lives in Southern California and loves to swim in the ocean. She will swim for miles because she loves being in the ocean. The feel and smell of the sea and nature compel her to engage in this form of physical entertainment. Only sharks and terribly cold water prevent her from getting into the ocean. So, when the ocean environment is not good, does she hustle down to a nearby pool and do laps for exercise? Absolutely not. It's just not the same. The pool laps are physical exercise, not physical entertainment.

In America, the number of outlets for true physical entertainment is very limited. With our huge, densely populated cities and our dependence on the automobile for our physical transportation needs, many of us suffer from a lack of physical entertainment opportunities. Too many of us are focused on balancing 50-hour-a-week jobs and ridiculously long commutes with our personal lives.

There's just doesn't seem to be any time left to force our exhausted bodies into the pay-for-use gyms that permeate our urban landscape—the gyms that focus on physical exercise, not physical entertainment. The problem with the current generation of pay-for-use gyms equipment is the focus. It's on physical exercise and not physical entertainment. Just think how a future anthropologist will dig up one of our StairMasters, NordicTracks, or Bowflex machines and wonder about its use. It must be some kind of torture machine. What else could it be?

But it's not all gloom and doom. I'm going to offer some suggestions on how the pay-for-use gyms could evolve their business model to physical entertainment and become more profitable. At the same time, many more Americans could experience the joy of physical entertainment.

But first, here's how I discovered the concept of physical entertainment. In 2002, I was extremely obese when I moved to the small community of Leadville, which is located in Lake County, Colorado. In 2012, Leadville was nationally rated second (Prescott, Arizona, was first) as a True Western Town by *True West* magazine.[3] I fell in love with the area because it is absolutely beautiful, and living here made me feel truly alive.

One of the county's crown jewels is the paved 12-mile Mineral Belt bike trail, which loops around the mining district. But I was too obese to ride my bike. I couldn't hike on the wonderful mountain trails that are everywhere. I couldn't ski at the nine world-class ski areas that are less than an hour's drive. I was too fat to bend over and fasten ski boots even if I could have found ski clothes that were big enough.

In March 2004, I began the long journey toward normal weight. Although there was a good indoor pool nearby, I wouldn't be seen dead in it because I was too fat and not thrilled at doing pool laps for exercise. So I didn't engage in any physical activity from March through May. But by June I had lost about 18 pounds, so I decided to try and get on my 20-year-old bike. With many stops and shaky legs, I finally completed the 12-mile loop around the Mineral Belt. I was completely exhausted but thrilled!

I got back on the bike again and again. It was during the long uphill climbs on the Mineral Belt trail that I began to question why I continued to get on my bike. The rides were physically very difficult, but I began to look forward to them. Why? Because the environment and scenery are stunning. As you slowly grind up the first six miles, you are able to see the beautiful trees, flowers, and occasional wildlife. You can smell the high mountain forest in all its glory. And the sun at 10,000 feet and the pure, dry air at 70 degrees are an experience that you cannot adequately describe. Then, as you swoop down the next six miles, you feel the cool, fresh mountain air on your skin and in your lungs. You feel truly alive. It was wonderful, and I came to feel deprived if the weather occasionally didn't cooperate. And the rides got easier and easier. Pretty soon I was pedaling that bike all the way around the 12-mile loop without stopping even once. In the process, I finally figured out that, for me, this was not physical exercise, but physical entertainment.

By late fall, I had lost almost 40 pounds. Since I live in Lake County, Colorado, where there are so many world-class ski areas within minutes, I decided to investigate the possibility of learning how to ski. Imagine my amazement to discover that the season pass prices for many of these ski areas are complete bargains! If you ski 50 days a year, the daily cost is only about $10!

So, in the fall of 2004, I decided I was going to take a huge risk and try to become a "real" skier. At age 53, it took a lot of courage for me to actually take this step in my life, because I didn't know how to ski. I went out and bought size extra-large ski clothing on sale and joined the nearby Copper Mountain On (Over) The Hill Gang for 50-plus-year-old skiers.[4] There was guided skiing, lessons, lots of emotional support, and many friendships to be found in Copper OHG. Once I learned how to ski and was not so afraid, I was able to experience the physical entertainment of skiing. I never have tried heroin or cocaine, but I am now addicted to another white powder. It's called snow.

So I don't exercise. But in my perfect world, there would be 100 days of perfect biking weather and 100 days of perfect snow conditions for skiing. That leaves 165 days to engage in some other form of physical entertainment or just not do anything at all.

Now, I've got some li'l old fat lady opinions on being physically active. Although I am now much more active that I have ever been in my entire life, I'm not convinced that physical activity equals significant, rapid, permanent weight loss. The first three months of my weight loss journey I was a couch potato. But I still lost about 18 pounds during that time. Then, at the tail end of my 90-pound weight loss journey, I had neck surgery. I was sidelined from doing any real physical activity for almost four months. But during that time, I still lost about four pounds, so I'm not sure that there's a direct correlation between physical activity and significant, rapid, permanent weight loss. But the data do seem to support the conclusion that modest daily physical activity can result in lower obesity rates. I'll cover this in more detail a little later.

That being said, I *am* convinced that physical activity offers significant benefits. In addition to health benefits, there's the physical aspect of losing lots of body mass. When I lost weight slowly and became physically active, all my body parts sort of went back where they were supposed to be. I didn't develop sagging this and hanging that. And here's another li'l old fat lady observation. When I was lugging around 90 extra pounds, my poor legs and back carried that strain. But those suckers had to be strong because they carried so much weight. By becoming active while I lost weight, I leveraged my extra muscle strength. So, I was at an advantage as I slowly lost weight. Why? Because having strong back and leg muscles really helped when I began to bike and ski.

Rather than just give you the opinions of a li'l old fat lady, here's what several doctors who specialize in diabetes and weight loss have to say. The first is from Dr. Richard K. Bernstein, MD, in his book *Dr. Bernstein's Diabetes Solution.*

> Although exercise does make weight control easier, it does not directly—at least not as much as we may wish—"burn fat." Unless you work out at very strenuous levels for several hours each day, exercise isn't going to have a significant direct effect upon your body fat. The effects of exercise are broader and more indirect. One of the great benefits is that many people find that when they exercise, they have less desire to overeat and are more likely to crave proteins than carbohydrates. The reasons for this are probably related to the release in the brain of neurotransmitters such as endorphins….It might be said that in the same way that obesity leads to further obesity, fitness leads to further fitness.[5]

And, here's what Dr. Stephen Phinney, MD, PhD, and Jeff Volek, PhD, RD, say in their new book, *The Art and Science of Low Carbohydrate Performance.*

> Why write this booklet now? What has changed is that we (not just the two of us, but the greater "we" encompassing many colleagues) are now wrapping up a remarkable decade of human research on diets lower in carbohydrate and commensurately higher in fats and protein. In the last 10 years, "we" have discovered that.
>
> • Low carbohydrate diets are anti-inflammatory, producing less oxidative stress during exercise and more rapid recovery between exercise sessions.
>
> • Physiological adaptation to low carbohydrate living allows much greater reliance on body fat, not just at rest but also during exer-

cise, meaning much less dependence on muscle glycogen and less need to reload with carbohydrates during and after exercise.

- Low carbohydrate adaption accelerates the body's use of saturated fats for fuel, allowing a high intake of total fats (including saturates) without risk.

- At the practice level, effective training for both endurance and strength/power sports can be done by individuals adapted to carbohydrate restricted diets, with desirable changes in body composition and power-to-weight ratios.[6]

Then there's Michael R. Eades, MD, and Mary Dan Eades, MD, who are physicians who specialize in weight loss, and they've written an excellent book, *Protein Power*, that I highly recommend. Even though they use that horrible word "exercise," these two medical doctors know what they're talking about. Here's what they have to say.

> Regular exercise plays an important role in helping you reclaim your health and vitality, not only in weight loss and maintenance, but also in lowered blood pressure and improved lipid values. More important even than that, dedication to regular physical exercise helps you milk all the pleasure you can from a long and healthy life. The goals of exercise are simple: increased muscle strength and endurance. Stronger, better-conditioned muscles lead to improved physical performance—not just in sporting endeavors, but in everyday activities. And best of all, exercise keeps you young! Although that may seem impossible, it's true; the right kind of exercise, coupled with the proper nutritional structure, will increase your release of growth hormone, that magic elixir of youth.[7]

Now, all we need to do is change our focus from physical exercise to physical entertainment and we will see a dramatic improvement in our lives. This li'l old fat lady has been there, done that, and it's absolutely true. Physical activity while I slowly lost weight helped me regain my health and vitality, too. Dr. Leder is convinced that my success at beating obesity, diabetes, and heart disease is partly due to becoming physically active while I slowly lost 90 pounds. But, if I hadn't focused on activities that are physical entertainment to me, it just wouldn't have happened. It's up to each of us to seek out and discover a few things in our lives that will get us to move a little every single day.

Although I choose to ride a bike and ski outdoors for physical entertainment, most communities in America don't have the enormous number of outdoor options that Lake County has, so maybe our pay-for-use gyms could fill that need. They could change their business model from being "sweat shops" to "physical entertainment spas." I'm talking about something that allows the poor, overworked, exhausted American to escape from reality for just a little while. Something that we would pay good money for and consider a luxury. With our current generation of computer technology, this is completely feasible.

Now, I know the dollar signs are blinking in neon colors, but it doesn't have to cost millions to get started. It doesn't have to cost very much money at all. The large cost here is forcing our brains to think outside-the-box to think of physical entertainment rather than physical exercise. Here are a few examples of low-cost ways to move in the right direction.

First, we could equip our existing "torture machines" with virtual reality that mimics the best of the outdoors. Here's an example. We put exercise bikes and/or bike trainers in a small room. In that room, we simulate the Leadville Mineral Belt Trail, both visually and environmentally. There's the sun, wind, temperature, and smell of this incredible place. You slowly climb six miles, savoring the beauty and scenery, and then careen six miles back down to your starting point. I bet you couldn't equip enough exercise bikes to satisfy the demand for this type of physical entertainment. I know I can never get enough of the real thing. And I would pay good money to be able to experience riding in other beautiful outdoor settings all over the world right in my local physical entertainment spa. Just provide me with a schedule of when and where we're riding, and I'll be there with my money.

Then, there are the StairMasters and NordicTracks…but I think you get the point. As time goes on and we get smarter about what constitutes physical entertainment for our customers, we can then begin to spend money on retrofitting our pay-for-use sweat shop gyms into really luxurious physical entertainment spas.

As an obese person, it was very hard to be active. I believe that water activities would have been the best option, since the water would have helped me achieve movement without putting excessive pressure on my joints or skeletal structure. But I wasn't about to try and put on one of those little skinny Speedo swim suits, even if they do make them in size 22. And I wasn't about to go hop in the pool with all those little kids or slim, athletic adults who were doing exercise laps in the pool. But if the pool had offered physical entertainment options for overweight and obese folks, I would have been in there just about every day.

So, what can you do in a pool besides laps? Well, when I was a kid, we used to throw coins into the pool and go dive after them. So maybe the pools could stock game pieces that could be checked out. Bending over in the shallow end of the pool to retrieve a game piece is an example of physical entertainment.

What about the possibility of tweaking yoga? While yoga is a beautiful, ancient, time-honored discipline, the marketers have recently gone into overdrive commercializing yoga in order to get us consumers to open our wallets. Many big-name clothing manufacturers have jumped on the yoga bandwagon. From Nike to Calvin Klein to prAna to North Face to Columbia Sportswear, yoga clothes really help with next quarter's earnings. Then there are the yoga mats, blocks, straps, balls, and even a thing called a Joby Gorillamobile Yogi iPad 2 Stand. And here are 14 different yoga varieties listed by *Women's Health* magazine.[7] Just take your pick. Anusara, Ashtanga, Bikram, Hatha, Lyengar, Jivamukti, Kripalu, Kundalini, Power, Prenatal, Restorative, Sivananda, Viniyoga, and Yin.

Let's take the example of "Bikram" yoga, also sometimes known as hot yoga. They say the heat and sweating are supposed to make you more limber and purify you, but I'm just not sold. It feels too much like physical exercise to me. I know someone who's a yoga instructor, and she does a beautiful job. But, the four times I went to a beginner class, the heat and humidity increased each time. So I told the yoga instructor that I just wasn't warming up to the heat. Regarding big money, according to *Women's Health* magazine, this style of yoga is called "Bikram" for inventor Bikram Choudhury. *Women's Health* magazine's website states, "The style is best-known for Choudhury's flamboyant capitalist shtick (he collects Bentleys and Rolls-Royces), outrageous quotes (I have b---- like atom bombs!), and Hollywood students (including the likes of Goldie Hawn)."[8] Yes, jumping onto the yoga bandwagon right now does mean big money.

I'm also convinced that the 200-million-plus Americans who are overweight or obese would have a difficult time doing a majority of the hot yoga poses, especially when the temperature and humidity are 105 degrees and 40%. But, with the aid of nice, cool water, maybe we could take some of the wonderful aspects of yoga and apply it to water yoga. I know, there are yoga purists who will cringe at this idea, but I don't believe that the original practitioners of yoga cranked up their furnaces and humidifiers to increase the heat and humidity. So, if we can embrace hot yoga, why can't we embrace water yoga?

Now, we don't want water yoga to be physical exercise, so maybe some soothing lights, music, and aroma could be added to increase the physical entertainment spa aspects of this physical activity. Maybe even some sort of virtual reality to simulate being on a beach in the South Pacific or somewhere else equally wonderful. How about some apres-water-yoga, pay-for-use amenities like mani-pedies, massages, hairdos, and skin treatments? Maybe a Starbucks type coffee lounge that has a "gold card" and offers delicious, rich, low PSS treats? And a designer boutique that carries attractive large-size water yoga clothes and special water yoga shoes? Watch out, I'm on a roll here.

Because water is such a good thing for overweight and obese folks, maybe we could create some water dance programs at our pools. Sort of like square dancing in water or whatever dance flavor that might turn physical exercise into physical entertainment. Or countless other water physical entertainment activities. The money-making opportunities in this area are limited only by our imaginations.

Now I realize I have lots of li'l old fat lady opinions, and you probably think that my ideas about being physically active in water are just my opinions, but they're not. Here's what the American College of Sports Medicine has to say:

> Despite the proven health benefits of aerobic exercise training, traditional modes, such as land walking and running, are often associated with an increased risk of musculosketetal injury due to accumulated stress on the lower extremities, particularly in the obese. Furthermore, pain and injury from exercise are often cited as reasons for discontinuing exercise training. To counter the joint injuries and orthopedic problems that often limit exercise in the obese, the ACSM recommends non-weight-bearing exercise for physical training in this population. In this regard, aquatic aerobic exercise reduces the stress on the lower extremities and spine and has been recommended for individuals who are overweight and who have orthopedic diseases, such as osteoarthritis. To date, however, few well-controlled studies have been published to quantify the effectiveness of aerobic water-based exercise training. Those that exist show that persons performing deep-water running, water walking, and aquatic dance training generally demonstrate similar improvements in aerobic capacity as those performing traditional land-based aerobic exercise training.[10]

But what about the large number of Americans who just aren't turned on by biking, skiing, and pools? I bet they're turned on about something. Most people have some form of entertainment outlet in their lives. We just need to turn on our brains to figure out what people enjoy doing and then create some way to turn that activity into physical entertainment.

Here's an example. I have a son-in-law who loves spectator sports. If it's football or baseball, he's hooked. He has my daughter rush out and purchase the latest football video game as soon as it's available for sale. But when he rips open the package and loads the game, what happens next? He sits down on the couch and exercises his thumbs. I've watched that video game and it's awesome. But, it would be wonderful if it provided just a little bit of physical entertainment opportunity. There could be various levels of physical activity offered so that anyone could participate although they might be very tired or obese. Even better would be physical entertainment spas that would feature spectator sports. Yes, I know that the Wii games sort of do this type of thing, but we need to create a total physical entertainment environment to get people to actually seek out this type of physical activity.

How about a bingo game that requires some sort of movement? Or a slot machine that moves more than one arm? We need to let our brains run wild, and I bet we can find some wonderful new ways to generate income for businesses and create physical entertainment opportunities for our poor, sick, obese citizens. America is known for its ingenuity, so I am certain we can crack this nut.

It would also be relatively inexpensive to design and install adult physical entertainment equipment in every existing park in America. While our children play on their swing sets and slides, we adults should be playing, too. Children don't exercise—they play. We need to take a lesson from our children.

Speaking of children, this li'l old fat lady didn't have an especially good experience as a child in PE. When I was in school, "PE" stood for physical education. If we could just get PE to stand for physical entertainment, I bet we could shift our focus from what is good for our children to what is pleasurable and fun. Maybe a little virtual reality wouldn't be a bad idea here, either.

Let me conclude this chapter by telling you a story. Colorado has 54 mountain peaks that are higher than 14,000 feet.[11] They're called 14ers, and almost half of the peaks are located within an hour of Lake County. About 25 years ago, I hiked a couple of the easier ones when I was normal weight. So I decided that I wanted to hike another one at the ripe old age of 60—it didn't even matter if it was the very easiest one, because the point was just to celebrate my freedom and health.

If you want an amazing hiking experience, hike up one of these 14ers—you will be on top of the world. Many of them are not technical, meaning that, if you can put hiking boots on, you can walk up them. But obesity is a problem if you want to successfully hike one of these 14,000-foot peaks. I spent hundreds of days skiing, rode thousands of miles on my bike, and shed 90 pounds before I successfully walked to the summit of one of these suckers.

At the summit of the 14er, the scenery was breathtaking, and my sense of accomplishment was sweet. I sat down on a rock to eat my low PSS snacks before I headed back down. As I rested, I overheard a normal-weight, middle-age woman telling her companions that she climbs 14ers so that she can eat chips and Pop-Tarts. I'm not joking, the woman said those exact words! That was the most difficult moment of my hike. It was almost impossible for me to keep my face straight and not hysterically laugh out loud. In order to eat our mainstream American foods and not become obese and sick, we need to climb 14,000-foot peaks. Isn't that just special!

CHAPTER 6

Your Best Friends Can Be Your Worst Enemies

You must be the change you want to see in the world.
—Mahatma Gandhi (1869–1948)

I have some of the best friends in the world. I met many of them when I lost 45 pounds and then learned how to ski. It's amazing how changing one thing for the better in your life can have a positive impact on other areas, too. When I met these folks, some of them were "wanna be" skiers like me. But, unlike most of my friends, I was still 45 pounds overweight when we began skiing together. Some of these friends were also into road biking. Biking up long, high-altitude mountain passes is challenging enough at normal weight on a good bike, but I was still 45 pounds overweight and had a 20-year-old bike. So I couldn't hope to keep up. After several years, I decided that enough was enough and it was time to finish my weight loss journey. That was when the trouble started.

Many of the friends I ski and bike with are either normal weight or below normal weight. They are not PSS sensitive like I am. Most of them are very "healthy" eaters, according to current diet doctrine. They eat copious quantities of organic carbs, very little if any meat, and avoid fat like the plague. They don't eat at fast food joints. And their dislike of fat is so bad that I would even use the term "pathologic revulsion." They almost spit when they utter the word. For these folks, "fat" is a four-letter word, so, in this chapter, I'm going to refer to "fat" as "phat!" Now, when you say the word, just spit it out.

Let me give you an example of "pathologic revulsion" of phat! Because I am so (reactive) hypoglycemic, I generally carry some sort of snack that is high in protein, fat, and fiber. If I feel my blood sugar start to drop, I just eat a few bites and everything is fine. My favorite snack is macadamia nuts, and Costco usually sells large cans of them at a very reasonable price. If I pull out my little snack bag of nuts, I will always offer it to my friends. One of my slightly underweight friends is so phat! phobic that she will allow herself to eat only one macadamia nut, even though she loves them. She carefully looks at the nuts in the bag and selects the biggest one since she can only have one. I think this behavior constitutes "pathologic revulsion" of phat!, don't you?

Now, I want to stress a point here. *Not once* have I ever tried to force my dietary beliefs on anyone else. When I am asked how I successfully and permanently lost so much weight, I've learned to say something like this: "The short answer is that I've eliminated almost all carbs." The people asking don't have a clue what I really mean. They think I mean dieting and restricting calories and phat!

But, my friends see what I eat, and a few of them just can't seem to control themselves. They have this compulsion to try and force their dietary beliefs on me. I'm not exaggerating. Because they truly care about me, they want to convert me to their brand of dietary religion. It is really hard for these folks to see me eat unhealthy phat! foods. And because they are not PSS sensitive like I am, they don't get fat eating PSS rich foods. They think they are thin because they are such "healthy" eaters. I believe they are thin because they are not PSS sensitive, and they restrict calories, protein, and phat! to the extreme.

Here is what I've learned by watching and listening. While many of these folks are exercise maniacs, normal weight, and eat healthy, organic, low phat! foods, the 60-plus-year-old ones still suffer from all sorts of ailments. Examples include diabetes, high cholesterol, high blood pressure, osteoporosis, arthritis, Parkinson's disease, and cancer. I'm the "black sheep" because I don't restrict calories and I eat a lot of protein and phat! I'm also not suffering from any of the diseases I just mentioned.

We fat folks are told we are fat because we don't eat right and don't get enough exercise. Right? Well, here's another interesting thing that I've learned. In addition to being "healthy eaters," most of my friends and acquaintances are exercise animals. Some of these folks do five-day, 350-mile bike rides over multiple 11,000-foot mountain passes. Others spend a month crossing Europe on a bicycle. A few are marathon runners, ski instructors, and yoga instructors. All of them are skiers. And almost all of them are frantically counting calories and restricting phat!

But they are still struggling to not gain weight even though they exercise like crazy, eat only healthy, organic foods, and restrict their phat! intake to the extreme. They think it's normal to be a slave to calorie restriction and phat! rationing. This has been their experience for most of their lives, so it feels like it's OK and normal to be a dietary hostage. They can't even see the long-term futility of constantly "renewing their vows" with Weight Watchers.

In my opinion, all of them are also carboholics. While they would vehemently deny it, they are addicted to high PSS foods. So, I believe that even these folks who are not PSS sensitive are suffering from the consequences of a high PSS diet.

Peggy Prediction: *One of these days I bet we're going to figure out that much of the "old person" weight gain that we attribute to a slowing metabolism is really due to our poor pancreas and insulin-resistant cells throwing in the towel after many decades of abuse.*

To help others who may decide to defy current diet doctrine, I'm going to relate a few of the worst experiences I've had during my weight loss journey. While these are not typical and most of my friends would never consider behaving this way, I believe that these examples can help you if you choose to defy current diet doctrine. Being prepared is the single best defense against dietary persecution from friends or family. So, here goes.

Just when I decided I was fed up with only being 45 pounds overweight rather than 90 pounds overweight, I had an opportunity to go cycling with two of my slightly underweight friends. The ride we took was a total of 40 miles, but it was pretty flat, so I could almost keep up. After 20 miles, we turned around and looked for a place to eat lunch. I brought one of my low-carb English muffins to eat. The other two ordered "healthy" high-carb sandwiches with fat-free dressings. When I started to eat my English muffin, I was interrogated. The conversation went like this. "So, Peggy, what's that you're eating?" I answered, "Just an English muffin." They asked, "So, what's on it?" I said, "Canadian bacon, gouda cheese, and Caesar salad dressing." The one asking the questions made a horrible face and said, "Oh my God, it's just full of phat!" I responded quietly, "Well, I've already lost 45 pounds eating this way." The response was, "Just imagine how much further you would be ahead if you ate right!" I was speechless. I didn't know how to respond. That was the moment this book was born.

Here's another example. Toward the end of my second 45-pound weight loss journey, I was at a party held at a friend's house. One person had contributed a wonderful-tasting, high-phat! dip. While I was helping myself to some, another friend commented that I shouldn't be eating the stuff. It was high phat! I responded that this was how I eat to lose weight. The friend's response was, "Well, we'll just see how much you weigh a year from now!" Well, it's been a year and the friend has become a mute. I guess they just can't admit that they were completely wrong.

Now, I'm going to describe the worst experience I ever had. It will illustrate just how bad things can get when friends and family members subscribe to a different dietary religion than you. In this country we value freedom of speech and religion, but, for some folks, that doesn't extend to what we eat.

I went with a number of friends on a weeklong vacation. There were two friends who apparently decided that this would be a good time to impose their dietary beliefs on me. With the zeal of religious zealots, they went after me. The week was spent in a very rural location, and we shared all of our meals. Only one of the friends was authorized to drive the rental car, so we all went to the grocery store as a group. We pooled our money to buy groceries, which was fine with me. But when I also tried to buy myself things like cheese, soy milk, and protein-rich foods, I was ridiculed and criticized repeatedly. I'm not exaggerating.

Then, at an open-air market, a vendor was offering rotisserie chicken. As I was attempting to buy myself some, one of the friends swooped over, shaking her head and exclaiming, "*Ooooh! That chicken is really greasy!*" The low-carb food items I brought with me were also targeted. Here's a comment that I received on my low-carb granola cereal: "This stuff has 12 grams of phat!"

During that week, there was not one meal served by any of my friends that contained significant amounts of protein and fat. Most of the food items were high PSS and included lots of bread, sugary desserts, and wine. After several days, I developed symptoms that resembled food poisoning, so one of my friends pulled out some medication that might help. I remember thinking that I definitely had food poisoning, but it wasn't the kind that they thought it was.

Because I had already decided to write this book, I chose to not resist this situation. If I had responded in an appropriate manner, the supply of amazing comments would have dried up. So, I meekly submitted to this completely inappropriate dietary situation in order to continue to gather more valuable book material.

I don't recommend you do the same. In the words of Apple founder Steven P. Jobs, "Don't let the noise of others' opinions drown out your own inner voice. And most important, have the courage to follow your heart and intuition."[1] Like with religion, some folks think they know all the answers, and they will put pressure on you to conform to their dietary beliefs. If you're right, then they must be wrong, and these people just can't cope with being wrong. So, here are my school-of-hard-knocks suggestions.

Never put yourself into a situation where anyone else can control what you eat. If someone invites you to be a guest in his or her house and then forces his or her dietary religion on you, you need to consider not accepting his or her invitation.

If someone feels that he or she has a right to impose his or her dietary religion on you, you need to politely but firmly reject his or her comments. A response along these lines would be appropriate: "I respect your dietary beliefs, and I ask that you please respect mine." Don't get into a justification of your beliefs, or an argument will ensue. Like with politics and religion, some people think they have all the right answers regarding what they eat.

Since calories, cholesterol, and phat! have been the darling demons for so many decades in America, the shift to high PSS foods becoming the darling demon will take lots of time. It's already taken lots of time—it's been almost 40 years since Dr. Robert C. Atkins was vilified and accused of being a fraud. So, if you choose to defy current diet doctrine like I did, just realize that lots of folks still think that the earth is at the center of the universe.

Don't argue with these people. Your friends or family members who still think that the earth is at the center of the universe can't hear what you have to say because it contradicts their fundamental dietary beliefs. And the more they care about you, the more they will attempt to make you conform to their beliefs.

At times it can be very hard to restrain yourself and keep your mouth shut. It becomes especially difficult when you realize that friends or family members are unwittingly contributing to their obesity and health problems by subscribing to the current dietary dogma that has plagued this country for the past 35 years. It can be overwhelming to hear of a sibling under the age of 50 who has stents, severe blockage of his heart, and crushing chest pain, or a parent in her 60s with type 2 diabetes who is having her eyes scraped. I've even know of folks with Medicare-age parents who must choose between an empty refrigerator and expensive prescription medicine that's required due to many decades of excessive carbohydrate consumption.

But your friends and family members who haven't figured out that the earth is not at the center of the universe can't turn the kaleidoscope. If you try and help them, all you will do is lose friends and alienate family members. Even if you don't impose your dietary beliefs on others, there will still be a few folks who become extremely insecure, uncomfortable, and mean. This is just how some folks deal with fundamental change. There's even a chance that you might lose a friend or two. But, if they're that small minded and myopic, were they ever really your friends or are they just a part of your social network?

There will be cases where folks inquire about how you achieved the elusive goal of significant weight loss and good health. Others will become secretly jealous of your success. A few will hope that you fail and make disparaging comments when your weight inevitably does one of its temporary backtracks. Here are the actual words that someone said to me when I was just a few pounds over my target goal weight, "Peggy, you're getting fat - looks like you're gaining weight!"

One mistake I made during my weight loss journey was to surround myself by too many thin friends who were not PSS sensitive. Not once have I ever been bashed by someone who truly struggled with their weight. So, there's this delicate balance between "running with the thin pack" and needing the emotional support from folks who "walk in your shoes."

I recommend you intentionally seek out folks from both extremes. The thin friends will inspire you to persevere and the not-so-thin ones will give you emotional support. Speaking of support, I don't like the organization name "Overeaters Anonymous." Most of the attendees are not guilty of gluttony but of carboholism. So, how about changing the name to Carboholics Anonymous? I realize there's a blog spot with this name, but it's just a blog. Overeaters Anonymous's website states that about 6,500 OA groups meet each week in over 75 countries.[2] This is the kind of support we need for carboholics.

Fortunately, there are a number of fledgling low PSS support resources. First, there's the Obesity Action Coalition that claims to be "the *only* national nonprofit whose sole focus is helping individuals affected by obesity." The OAC website is: *www.obesityaction.org*. In addition to providing good information, OAC says it's also working to become active on state-based legislative and regulatory activities. My only beef with the OAC is the first sentence on their bariatric (weight-loss) surgery page, which states, "Weight-loss surgery is a safe and effective treatment option for those affected by severe obesity."[3] This li'l old fat lady suspects some the families and loved ones of the thousands of bariatric surgery patients who have died might disagree with this statement.

Then, there's Jimmy Moore. In addition to his two inspirational books, *Livin' La Vida Low-Carb* and *21 Life Lessons from Livin' La Vida Low-Carb*, Jimmy is an energy power-house who has managed to put together an amazing collection of valuable information on his websites. The information ranges from excellent podcasts several times a week to a growing list of physicians in nearly all 50 states willing to use a healthy, low-carb, nutritional approach. If a physician is a member of the American Society of Bariatric Physicians (www.asbp.org) *and* is a member of the Nutrition and Metabolism Society (www.nmsociety.org) *and* is on Jimmy's physician list, chances are very good that you'll get the help you need. I call Jimmy Moore the *Consumer Reports* of low carb. He's also a wonderful cheerleader.

Here's what Jimmy's website says: "In January 2004, Jimmy Moore made a decision to get rid of the weight that was literally killing him. At 32 years of age and 410 pounds, the time had come for a radical change of lifestyle. A year later, he had shed 180 pounds, shrunk his waist by 20 inches, and dropped his shirt size from 5XL to XL. After his dramatic weight loss, Jimmy was inundated with requests from friends, neighbors, and complete strangers seeking information and help. Jimmy is dedicated to helping as many people as possible find the information they need to make the kind of lifestyle change he has made. To that end, he has started a blog and a number of websites to get out the message of lifestyle change and healthy living." Jimmy's main website is: *www.livinlavidalowcarb.com*. You'll be happy you checked it out.

Next, there's the website *www.CarbSmart.com* that recently transitioned from online retailer to online information source. "Providing low-carb products is only the first half of the equation to winning the war with obesity," says company founder and president Andrew DiMino. "The second half is helping people obtain reliable information, so they can make educated, informed choices about which products are best for them, how to make the right diet choices, and how to easily make the low-carb lifestyle part of their daily lives, even when they're working or on vacation." *CarbSmart.com* managing editor Dana Carpender, who is also a best-selling low-carb cookbook author and columnist, says, "We're expanding our focus to cover such topics as how to be successful on a low-carb diet and how to control or eliminate diabetes." During its 13-year history, CarbSmart has helped nearly 15 million people worldwide benefit from and adopt the low-carb lifestyle. "We've helped people from all walks of life learn how to eat healthier and achieve their ideal weight the low-carb way," says DiMino.

Last, but not least, there's the website *www.dietdoctor.com*. This blog is hosted by Andreas Eenfeldt, MD, who is a Swedish medical doctor specializing in family medicine. Dr. Eenfeldt is a strong advocate of the low-carb dietary philosophy, and his blog has a completely amazing library of video clips. Many of his videos feature fellow medical doctors, including Richard K. Bernstein, MD; Michael R. Eades, MD; Michael D. Fox, MD; Robert H. Lustig, MD (recently featured on *60 Minutes*); Dr. Stephen D. Phinney, MD, PhD; Mary C. Vernon, MD; Eric C. Westman, MD; and Dr. Jay Wortman, MD. All these MDs are "big dogs" when it comes to understanding the medicine behind low carb.

Organizations and websites like these can provide essential support to help us with our carbohydrate addictions, and I wish more had existed as I went through my weight loss journey. Instead, many times I would just muddle my way along until I came up with a solution that worked. Let me bare my soul and tell you about my most challenging carbohydrate addiction.

No, it wasn't chocolate, chips, or ice cream. It was red wine. Not white wine, hard liquor, or beer. Only red wine. And only for a little while late in the afternoons. While I was at the 230-plus-pounds mark, I could put an entire 750 milliliter bottle of red wine away and toddle off to sleep. The next morning, I would feel great. I know that red wine is supposed to be relatively low in carbohydrates. Even Dr. Bernstein's *Diabetes Solution* says, "Ethyl alcohol, which is the active ingredient in hard liquor, beer, and wine, has no direct effect on blood sugar because the body does not convert it into glucose."[4] But my ornery pancreas doesn't buy it. I'm not sure why, but within moments of the first sip, my blood sugar appears to experience a dramatic rise, and that sensation of pleasure is truly addictive. I realize we separate carbohydrates from alcohol on the nutrition labels, but the primary ingredients in red wine are water, grapes, and sugar. Grapes and sugar will both kick my pancreas into overdrive.

Bees don't buy it either. Bees are always attracted to sugars and, if there's sugar in something, they'll go after it. Someone I know makes a lot of homemade wine and she'll take the "mash" that contains the pulp of the grapes in the wine and put it in the compost outside. Then the bees will swarm the "mash" and proceed to become drunk. It is extremely funny to watch a drunk bee try and fly straight. They behave just like us humans when we've been hitting the sauce. So, yes, this li'l old fat lady believes that, for some unknown reason, my pancreas perceives wine and other alcohols as a high PSS. And, from hard-earned experience, I know that regularly drinking even small amounts of red wine too often will send my weight in the wrong direction. It's not just this li'l old fat lady's opinion either. Alcohol was on Dr. Leder's "no-no" list, and Michael R. Eades, MD, and Mary Dan Eades, MD, recommend not drinking every day, even when your weight is normal.[5]

I finally overcame my physical, metabolic addiction to red wine by figuring out that my blood sugar predictably drops just about every day in the late afternoon. The secret is to not let this happen. Macadamia nuts (or some other low PSS high protein snack) and a cup of half decaffeinated, half caffeinated coffee prevents this nasty drop in blood sugar. No blood sugar drop results in no red wine craving. No red wine craving results in no caving.

Because I am an ornery old cuss, I still drink a small amount of red wine on occasion. It's always at parties (along with other things I don't normally eat) but I don't drink very much wine anymore because two glasses of the stuff will now cause a major hangover. I still don't keep red wine in my house because I'll always find an excuse to drink it. That's the way it is with carbohydrates and other addictions. Would I consider myself to be an alcoholic? Here's what I stated earlier: "Someone who consumes alcohol to the point of negative consequences is an alcoholic." So my response is—yes! Now, I want to emphasize this point. Some folks can't drink alcoholic beverages at all. One serving of anything will set them up for failure. If you're one of these individuals, just don't do it.

Peggy Prediction: *Almost all alcoholics are also carboholics. A low PSS diet could help eliminate some of the alcoholism we have in this country.*

We each need to take responsibility for searching out individual solutions that will allow us to succeed as we go through life. Being addiction free allows us to experience life to the fullest. This includes *all* addictions, not just alcohol, tobacco, and illegal drugs. Yes, it can be terribly difficult to break free, but the joy of success is immense. It is definitely worth every bit of the frustration and self-searching necessary to successfully come out the other side. Yes, it can be done, and the rewards are absolutely huge. But, like all addictions, the abnormal wiring in our brains will continue to make us crave comfort foods and sweets. That's why I have my cake and eat it too.

While I have focused primarily on how to manage friends and acquaintances, here's an enlightening and entertaining editorial written by Dana Carpender, managing editor of *CarbSmart.com*, that speaks to holiday occasions and problem family members. Dana is also a prolific low-carb-cookbook author—I own six of her books and can attest to how great they are. In addition to wearing all of her other hats, she also regularly blogs at her website, *www.HoldtheToast.com*.

Posted October 30, 2010

It's Halloween weekend, and you know what that means: the holidays are straight ahead, and with them piles and piles of carby junk, and worse, people nagging you to eat the stuff. Why so many people think that saying things like "But you have to eat it! It's traditional!" and "I worked all afternoon making it just for you" constitutes an expression of holiday goodwill, I have no idea, but sadly this behavior is all too common. You need to think ahead about how to respond to this sort of thing.

You have absolutely no obligation to eat anything you do not want to eat. If you had a terrible allergy, the sort that would throw you into anaphylaxis at the merest taste, you would not hesitate to refuse that food, nor would you apologize for doing so. Similarly, if you were a re-covering alcoholic, you would feel free to say "No, thanks," to a drink, and would consider rude anyone who pressed you. Carbohydrate ad-diction and hyperinsulinemia don't kill as quickly as allergic reactions, but they kill vastly more people, and a case can be made that dying quickly of anaphylaxis is preferable to the long, drawn-out years of deteriorating health and increasing debility that carb addiction can wreak on the body.

So no feeling apologetic. When offered food or drink one does not care to consume, "No, thank you" is always a polite thing to say. Conversely, nagging people to eat foods they have politely refused is rude-rude-rude. You are in the right here, no matter how people try to browbeat you into thinking you're the unmannerly one.

Do not JADE: Justify, Argue, Defend, or Explain. Do you really want to bore everyone at the table with a stirring defense of low carbohydrate diets, complete with medical journal citations? Heck, no, it's just not festive.

More importantly, any explanation or justification past "No, thank you" or "I don't care for any, thanks" will be seized upon as an op-portunity to argue with your decision. You've heard this sort of thing:

You: "No, thanks, I'm on a diet." Them: "Nobody diets on Christmas!"

You: "No, thanks, I'm avoiding carbs." Them: "That crazy diet! Everyone knows it's unhealthy. You're killing yourself! Come on, you have to have some!"

Etc. Every good salesman works to get the hesitant prospect to state his objections - because that's the moment he can start arguing them away. Do not let yourself in for this. YOU DO NOT NEED A REASON BEYOND "I don't care for any, thanks." You just don't.

However, it can be hard not to embellish on "No, thank you." So instead of offering an explanation or a defense, change the subject. Like this:

Them: "Oh, you have to try my famous cornbread stuffing!" You: "No, thank you. Hey, what's playing at the local movie theater? Is RED still there? I've been wanting to see it."

Let's try it again:

Them: "You haven't had any banana bread! I used great-grandma's recipe. You have to have some!" You: "No, thank you. By the way, does anyone want to go shopping tomorrow? I hear there's a huge sale at Macy's."

You get the idea. If you know that you're going to be confronted with busybodies and nags, practice this in advance. Come up with a list of conversation-changers. "What do you want for Christmas?" "Has anyone heard from Uncle Bill recently?" "Can you believe how our football team is doing?" "I got the coolest new app for my phone the other day, you've got to see it!" "When does Junior's holiday break start?" Anything will do, really.

What this does is make it far, far harder for the person shoving the food at you to continue. If you only say "No, thank you," you're going to hear "But you must have some!" and it's going to turn into a whole back-and-forth tug-o-war - "I don't want to." "But you have to!" "But I don't want to." "But you have to!" Argh. But once you've said "Hey, have you seen cousin Suzy's new house?" or whatever, the food-pusher is going to look just a tad obsessed if she keeps going. Instead of the other diners looking at you funny, they're going to look at the food-pusher funny. It's a neat form of social ju-jitsu.

One tangential but related tactic: If you come from a family where holiday get-togethers are an occasion to be "honest" - in other words, for people to say unkind things to one another - arm yourself with my all-purpose comeback: "How very kind of you to say so."

Again, let's practice:

"You've been on that diet for six months now, and you're still fat." "How very kind of you to say so."

"Haven't you gotten married yet? You're not getting any younger, you know." "How very kind of you to say so."

"Your sister just got a promotion. Thank heaven ONE of my children amounts to something." "How very kind of you to say so."

Isn't this fun? You're driving the thrower-of-darts out of their flippin' mind, and making him or her look like an ass, all while remaining impeccably polite.

Next year, have dinner with friends.

© 2010 by Dana Carpender. Used by permission of the author.

OK, enough laughing—now, let's get serious for a moment. This li'l old fat lady believes that the next few decades in America will see a dramatic shift from the old dietary dogma to an age of nutritional enlightenment. So, those of us who choose to defy current diet doctrine will suffer less and less as time goes on. But, obese ill folks like me can't wait. We must find the courage to occasionally suffer from dietary prosecution so that we can regain our personal freedom and health. We must each decide for ourselves that we are fed up with our current situation before we can turn the kaleidoscope to see beyond the old dietary dogma that has made Americans so obese and unhealthy. But we need to see what *can* be rather than what *is*. We need to be able to raise ourselves above the ideas of the time.

Your greatest argument in favor of your dietary religion is you. By successfully losing excess weight and becoming completely healthy, you present a very compelling argument in favor of your dietary beliefs. In the words of Gandhi, "You must be the change you want to see in the world."

CHAPTER 7

Where You Live Can Make a Difference

The pressure-sensitive adhesive used in 3M's famous Post-it Notes languished from 1968 to 1980. It can take a long time for a good idea to catch on.—Peggy June Forney

While the foundation for our personal freedom and health is based on eating low PSS foods, where we live can also impact our chances for success. I've included this chapter to help both obese, sick individuals and struggling businesses understand that geography can also play a role. Although many folks would never consider moving away from their friends or children, this information can still help you devise strategies to improve your situation.

You may disagree with some of my li'l old fat lady conclusions, but the underlying data sources are pristine. All of them are available on the Internet and can be accessed with a few keystrokes. Now, if you will turn the kaleidoscope, you can see what this li'l old fat lady is seeing. So, look at the numbers—they tell a very powerful story.

As a general rule, people who live where there are lots of natural amenities weigh less, have less diabetes, and are more physically active than people who live where there are few natural amenities. On average, they also live longer. How do I know this? Because I matched up data from a number of US government sources and research organizations that clearly shows this correlation. Let's start with these two government sources.

1. A 1999 United States Department of Agriculture (USDA) natural amenities scale that ranks all counties in the lower 48 states for natural amenities.[1] The report does not include Alaska, Hawaii, or Puerto

Rico. Each county in the lower 48 states is ranked according to natural amenities such as climate, topography, and water area that reflect environmental qualities most people prefer. These measures are warm winter, winter sun, temperate summer, low summer humidity, topographic variation, and water area. The total number of USDA-ranked counties is 3,111, with number one ranked highest and 3,111 ranked lowest for natural amenities.

2. The Centers for Disease Control (CDC) data that track obesity, diabetes, and physical inactivity rates at the county level.[2] The most recent year posted is 2009. In addition to the lower 48 states, the CDC data also include five Hawaii counties and 29 Alaska boroughs and areas. Since the 1999 USDA report, Colorado also added one more county. So, the final CDC total of counties is 3,146.

Here's an average of the fifty lowest-obesity-rated counties compared to the fifty highest-obesity-rated counties. The average rates of obesity, diabetes, and lack of physical activity are more than 200% higher in counties that have fewer natural amenities compared to those counties with more natural amenities.

AVERAGE OBESITY	AVERAGE AMENITY RANKING	AVERAGE % OBESITY	AVERAGE % DIABETES	AVERAGE % INACTIVE
50 LOWEST Obesity Counties	283 (high) out of 3,111	17.3%	5.4%	15.8%
50 HIGHEST Obesity Counties	1,843 (low) out of 3,111	41.2% (238% higher)	13.9% (257% higher)	34.3% (217% higher)

Colorado dominates the fifty lowest-obesity-rated counties with twenty-nine counties. Mississippi, with sixteen counties and Alabama, with eleven counties, dominate the fifty highest-obesity-rated counties. Here are the statistics for the two counties with the lowest and highest obesity rates in the country. The rates of obesity, diabetes, and lack of physical activity are 336%–426% higher in the county that has fewer natural amenities.

COUNTY & STATE	AMENITY RANKING	% OBESITY	% DIABETES	% INACTIVE
Routt County, CO	90 (high)	13.5%	3.8%	11.1%
Green County, AL	1,472 (low)	47.9% (355% higher)	16.2% (426% higher)	37.3% (336% higher)

Now, I'm going to show you the top 50 counties and the bottom 50 counties listed in order of obesity rates. Once you have an opportunity to look over the two lists, I'll then draw some 'lil old fat lady conclusions that are based on the data.

TOP 50 COUNTIES LISTED BY INCREASING OBESITY RATE
(High Amenity Ranking = Low Number)

STATE	COUNTY	AMENITY RANKING	% OBESITY	% DIABETES	% INACTIVE
CO	ROUTT	90	**13.5**	3.8	11.1
WY	TETON	87	**13.8**	4.4	10.6
CO	EAGLE	156	**13.9**	4.2	11.8
NM	SANTA FE	307	**14.1**	3.9	12
CO	PITKIN	54	**14.2**	4.7	12.7
CO	BOULDER	71	**14.5**	4.6	11.3
CA	MARIN	18	**15**	5.4	12.1

CO	SUMMIT	19	**15.1**	4.7	12.3
NY	NEW YORK	1684	**15.2**	7.2	16.4
CO	DOUGLAS	104	**15.7**	4.6	11.1
CO	GUNNISON	132	**15.7**	4.8	15.3
UT	SUMMIT	131	**15.7**	4.5	13
CO	CHAFFEE	47	**15.9**	4.6	15.6
CO	LA PLATA	69	**15.9**	4.6	15.5
CO	SAN MIGUEL	108	**16.4**	5.4	13.7
CO	ARCHULETA	80	**16.5**	5	16.7
CO	OURAY	57	**17**	5.4	15
NY	WESTCHESTER	915	**17**	6.7	18.6
CA	SAN FRANCISCO	6	**17.2**	7.3	17
CO	CONEJOS	123	**17.2**	4.7	18.9
ID	BLAINE	318	**17.2**	5.3	13.3
CO	GARFIELD	214	**17.3**	5.4	15.5
MT	GALLATIN	210	**17.4**	4.4	17.3

CO	CLEAR CREEK	37	**17.7**	5.1	17.3
CO	LAKE	11	**17.7**	5.1	18.9
CO	PARK	33	**17.7**	5	19.2
CO	TELLER	52	**17.8**	6	18.7
CT	FAIRFIELD	422	**18**	5.8	19.2
MA	BARNSTABLE	594	**18.1**	6.1	16.6
MD	MONTGOMERY	1862	**18.1**	6.5	16.6
CO	DENVER	324	**18.2**	6.1	16.3
MA	DUKES	322	**18.2**	7.8	18.1
CO	GRAND	25	**18.3**	5.2	16.9
CO	LARIMER	77	**18.5**	5	14.2
CO	MONTROSE	316	**18.6**	4.9	18.9
CO	JEFFERSON	79	**18.7**	5.2	15.7
CO	MINERAL	72	**18.7**	5.2	17.2
CO	SAN JUAN	31	**18.8**	5.3	18.4
NM	LOS ALAMOS	305	**18.8**	5.3	14.4

NM	TAOS	189	**18.8**	5.9	15.7
CO	HINSDALE	38	**18.9**	5.3	18.3
CO	MONTEZUMA	167	**18.9**	5.7	19.8
CO	GILPIN	36	**19.2**	5.4	18.7
WA	SAN JUAN	172	**19.2**	4.9	13.1
CO	ARAPAHOE	399	**19.4**	5.8	17.2
FL	MONROE	59	**19.4**	6.1	18.1
VA	ARLINGTON	2676	**19.4**	7.5	17.6
CA	SANTA CRUZ	12	**19.5**	6.1	12.4
CT	LITCHFIELD	798	**19.7**	6.1	18.5
CA	SAN MATEO	17	**19.8**	6.5	16.1

BOTTOM 50 COUNTIES LISTED BY INCREASING OBESITY RATE
(Low Amenity Ranking = High Number)

STATE	COUNTY	AMENITY RANKING	% OBESITY	% DIABETES	% INACTIVE
AL	RUSSELL	1630	**39.5**	12.5	36.5
MS	JASPER	2197	**39.5**	14.4	35.5
ND	ROLETTE	2660	**39.5**	13.3	35.4
OH	LAWRENCE	2187	**39.5**	11.3	35.4
KY	BREATHITT	2305	**39.6**	14.7	33.7
MS	WALTHALL	2053	**39.6**	12.4	34.9
SC	CALHOUN	1314	**39.6**	12.9	32.8
AR	PHILLIPS	1930	**39.7**	13.2	37.8
MD	SOMERSET	1477	**39.7**	11.4	32
MS	GREENE	1423	**39.7**	12.1	32.7
MS	WILKINSON	1521	**39.7**	14.9	35.3
NC	EDGECOMBE	2633	**39.7**	12.1	30.4
SC	JASPER	1026	**39.7**	12.9	30.2

MI	SAGINAW	2973	**39.9**	9.8	30.2
MS	NOXUBEE	1154	**39.9**	13.7	33.4
MS	PIKE	1665	**39.9**	13.7	35.2
KY	LINCOLN	2265	**40.1**	11.7	37.8
MS	QUITMAN	2576	**40.1**	15.1	34.8
MS	SHARKEY	2298	**40.2**	13.3	35.2
MS	TUNICA	1758	**40.2**	14.2	39.1
AL	MARENGO	1960	**40.4**	14.8	34.8
AL	PERRY	893	**40.5**	17.8	34.1
MS	COVINGTON	2196	**40.7**	12	30.8
MS	HOLMES	2085	**40.8**	14.1	35.3
NC	ROBESON	2392	**40.9**	13.3	38.5
SD	SHANNON	1534	**40.9**	16.8	32.4
SC	ORANGEBURG	1259	**41**	13.5	32.2
SD	TODD	2122	**41**	14.4	31.5
SC	HAMPTON	1940	**41.1**	14.3	30

SD	BUFFALO	2425	**41.2**	17.2	36.8
AL	BUTLER	2221	**41.3**	14.6	35.9
MS	HUMPHREYS	2227	**41.4**	13.6	33.4
MS	SUNFLOWER	2365	**41.4**	14.4	34.6
SC	BAMBERG	1977	**41.5**	12.6	33.1
MS	CLAIBORNE	1717	**41.6**	14.5	39.9
AL	MACON	1853	**41.7**	14.2	31.1
SD	CORSON	1956	**41.7**	13	31.6
ND	SIOUX	2112	**41.8**	13.5	32.3
AL	DALLAS	1584	**41.9**	14.2	33.3
SC	WILLIAMSBURG	2063	**41.9**	13.4	31.4
SD	DEWEY	1013	**42.3**	15.5	33.9
AL	SUMTER	1806	**42.4**	16.8	32.3
SC	MARLBORO	1243	**42.7**	12.7	33.1
SD	ZIEBACH	1848	**43.3**	14.1	34.5
AL	HALE	625	**43.5**	14	35.2

AL	WILCOX	575	**43.6**	15.5	34.4
MS	COAHOMA	1915	**44.3**	14.7	36.1
AL	LOWNDES	1764	**44.7**	16.4	37.5
MS	JEFFERSON	1953	**44.9**	15.3	37.2
AL	GREENE	1472	**47.9**	16.2	37.3

OK, it's time to draw some conclusions from all these numbers. You may disagree with me because some of them are just li'l old fat lady conclusions, but I have a really good track record for being right on this kind of stuff. So I challenge the scientists and statisticians to prove me wrong.

Now, either the folks living in the low natural amenity places are badder and worser than the folks living in the high natural amenity places, or something else in going on. I'm betting that something else is going on, so here's the li'l old fat lady's explanation. This is going to take a while, because there's a lot going on.

Mother Nature dictates that most of us do things that are pleasurable. So, when the outdoor environment stinks, most people turn into couch potatoes. Ditto when they're obese. When you've got obesity and physical inactivity, you've got diabetes and vice versa. When you eat a high PSS diet and live in a low natural amenity place, lots of folks get all three—obesity, diabetes, and physical inactivity. You also get a significantly shorter life expectancy.

So, in low natural amenity states like Mississippi and Alabama, we need to aggressively offer low PSS food options and get the physical exercise industry to start offering more in the way of physical entertainment opportunities. Yes, I know the 2010 Census shows that Mississippi has a black population of 37.3% and Alabama has a black population of 26.5%, but we need to stop using race and gender as excuses for our obesity epidemic.

Since there are 27 counties in these two states with the worst obesity rates in the country, we need to have lots of pools and lots of physical entertainment programs that involve pools. I know pools cost money, but obesity cost us Americans about $147 billion extra in medical care costs in 2008.[3] If the current obesity trend continues, that number is projected to be about $861 billion to $957 billion by 2030.[4] By spending a little money now on low PSS food options and pools, we can save a whole lot of money down the road. We can also prevent lots of unnecessary suffering and premature deaths.

Still not convinced that where you live makes a difference? Well, let's look at Colorado. Colorado is the leanest state in the country, with 29 of the 50 leanest counties. So 45% of Colorado's 64 counties are in the top 50 from a low obesity standpoint. The average natural amenity ranking of these 29 counties is 104 (high) out of 3,111 (low). So, there is a big correlation between high natural amenities and low rates of obesity, diabetes, and physical inactivity.

But if natural amenities were the whole story, California should win the low obesity game. When you rank the lower 48 states by natural amenities, California has the top 10 counties in the country, and 30 of the top 50 counties. In comparison, Colorado only has 10 counties in the top 50 when ranked by natural amenities. Here's the list of the top 50 counties ranked by natural amenities.

TOP 50 COUNTIES RANKED BY NATURAL AMENITY
(High Amenity Ranking = Low Number)

STATE	COUNTY	AMENITY RANKING	% OBESITY	% DIABETES	% INACTIVE
CA	VENTURA	1	22.9	6.8	16.8
CA	HUMBOLDT	2	25.9	8.1	18.9
CA	SANTA BARBARA	3	19.9	6.6	15.8
CA	MENDOCINO	4	22.6	6.3	17

CA	DEL NORTE	**5**	27.2	7.6	18.1
CA	SAN FRANCISCO	**6**	17.2	7.3	17
CA	LOS ANGELES	**7**	21.4	7.7	18.9
CA	SAN DIEGO	**8**	22.8	7.3	17.4
CA	MONTEREY	**9**	22.3	7.3	16
CA	ORANGE	**10**	20.5	7.1	16.4
CO	LAKE	**11**	17.7	5.1	18.9
CA	SANTA CRUZ	**12**	19.5	6.1	12.4
CA	CONTRA COSTA	**13**	24.2	6.9	17.3
CA	CALAVERAS	**14**	25.6	6.7	19.3
CA	MARIPOSA	**15**	24.1	7.2	19.4
CA	MONO	**16**	20.3	6.5	13.6
CA	SAN MATEO	**17**	19.8	6.5	16.1
CA	MARIN	**18**	15	5.4	12.1
CO	SUMMIT	**19**	15.1	4.7	12.3
CA	SONOMA	**20**	22.7	6.1	14.2

CA	SAN LUIS OBISPO	**21**	21.5	5.9	14.2
NV	DOUGLAS	**22**	21.7	6.3	16.4
CA	NAPA	**23**	22.1	6.2	15.1
AZ	GILA	**24**	26.5	8.7	23.1
CO	GRAND	**25**	18.3	5.2	16.9
CA	ALPINE	**26**	24.9	7.9	19.4
NV	CARSON CITY	**27**	23.1	7.1	19.8
CA	NEVADA	**28**	20.1	5.5	12.9
CA	AMADOR	**29**	24.8	8	16.6
CA	STANISLAUS	**30**	30.2	8.2	23.9
CO	SAN JUAN	**31**	18.8	5.3	18.4
AZ	COCHISE	**32**	23.8	7.2	22.3
CO	PARK	**33**	17.7	5	19.2
CA	TUOLUMNE	**34**	23.1	6	18.1
CA	INYO	**35**	23.1	6.9	16.7
CO	GILPIN	**36**	19.2	5.4	18.7

CO	CLEAR CREEK	37	17.7	5.1	17.3
CO	HINSDALE	38	18.9	5.3	18.3
OR	DOUGLAS	39	31.3	9.2	20.6
NV	WASHOE	40	22.6	6.4	17.2
NM	SIERRA	41	26.5	6.1	24.3
CA	RIVERSIDE	42	27.5	8.9	21.5
CA	LAKE	43	26.5	7.8	16.6
CA	PLUMAS	44	23.9	6.6	18.4
WA	CLALLAM	45	28.4	8.2	17.6
OR	CURRY	46	30.2	7.6	21.6
CO	CHAFFEE	47	15.9	4.6	15.6
CA	IMPERIAL	48	24.6	7.3	22.6
CO	JACKSON	49	20.5	5.4	17.9
NM	GRANT	50	23.8	6	19.2

Again, California has the top 10 counties in the country, and 30 of the top 50 counties. Colorado has only 10 counties in the top 50. If natural amenities were the whole story, California should win the low obesity game. So, why isn't California the leanest state in the country? Well, this li'l old fat lady believes that there is another variable operating in Colorado.

Peggy Prediction: *Coloradoans are leaner than the rest of the country partly because they're higher. Not drugs or alcohol high. Altitude high.*

Now, before you dispatch the straitjacket team and commit me to the insane asylum, please give me a chance to tell you why I believe that altitude may have an impact on our weight. When I moved to Lake County, Colorado, in 2002, I was extremely obese and quickly noticed that there were relatively few fatties like me. There should be lots of obese people living here. Why? Because Lake County houses many of the Hispanic resort workers who work in the large, rich, ski resort towns next door in Summit and Eagle Counties. According to the *Journal of the American Medical Association*, the obesity rate for Hispanics is 38.7% compared to 32.4% for whites.[5] Since the 2010 US Census data indicate that Lake County's population consists of 39.9% Hispanics, this county should be swarming with obese people. Right? Well, it's not. There are relatively few obese people living in this county.

Let's take a closer look. With a ranking of 11 out of 3,111, Lake County is the highest natural amenity rated county in Colorado. The large majority of the population lives in or near the city of Leadville, the highest incorporated city in the country with an elevation of 10,152 feet. Even with the 39.9% Hispanic population, the CDC estimates that the obesity rate for Lake County is only 17.7%.

So, why do I think that altitude is a factor? Because a crusty old man told me about the effect that altitude has on combustion engines. Here's the story. I was thinking about buying a little 6,500-watt generator to temporarily provide electricity to my property, and that crusty old man snickered loudly at this stupid li'l old fat lady. He told me a 6,500-watt generator would be worthless at 10,000 feet because the altitude significantly decreases the generator's power. I thought he was just playing games with this li'l old fat lady.

But when I checked out his story, I found that he was indeed correct. Here's the deal. Each motor/engine/furnace will react differently, but a general rule of thumb is that for every 1,000 feet of altitude increase, anything combustion loses approximately 3% of its power. At 10,000 feet, that's 30%. Lots of civilian and military aircraft fly in and out of the Lake County Airport. Sometimes there are strange-looking cars on the road with their identities concealed, bearing Michigan license plates. They're all conducting high altitude performance testing. And all the furnaces I put in the seven homes I built in

Lake County were significantly "derated" for the altitude. That means a bigger furnace is required to adequately heat the square footage of a given size house.

So, this li'l old fat lady's logic says that although we humans aren't machines, we still metabolize foods a little like machines. Maybe we humans have to work 30% harder at 10,000 feet than at sea level to just breathe and move? The lower birth weights of babies born at this altitude have been studied extensively, but there's a pathetic lack of research regarding the effects of high altitude on obesity.

An April 4, 2010, study titled *Hypobaric Hypoxia Causes Body Weight Reduction in Obese Subjects* states, "This study shows that obese subjects lose weight at high altitudes."[6] The study was done by scientists and researchers located in Munich, Germany. Why wasn't that study done here in America? We're the country with the catastrophic obesity problem. We've already got a Colorado Center for Altitude Medicine and Physiology. So, maybe this center or some other research organization could do something really outside-the-box and see if sleeping eight hours a night in an environment that simulates high altitude will help obese people lose weight. I know this idea sounds ridiculous, but the idea of eating lots of calories, fat, and protein to lose 90 pounds and become completely healthy also sounds ridiculous. At least to folks who subscribe to the old dietary dogma of "a calorie is a calorie."

I'm not the only one who's contemplating outside-the-box things to do while people sleep. There are respectable scientists conducting research in this area. Here's an example. In a study, *Mechanisms of Obesity-Induced Male Infertility*, one of three biological mechanisms linking obesity to impaired male reproductive function is "testicular heat stress/hypoxia-induced apoptosis." The scientific study authors state, "Testicular heat stress may be alleviated through increased activity, weight loss, and use of air-cooling devices during sleep."[7] You never know, given our exploding obesity epidemic, maybe those little bed fans will become a real money maker.

And here's another outside-the-box study from the scientific community regarding insulin control. It's titled *Exenatide: From the Gila Monster to the Pharmacy*. This one involves gila monster spit. "Exenatide offers a wide range of beneficial glucoregulatory effects, including enhancement of glucose-dependent insulin secretion, restoration of first-phase insulin response, suppression of inappropriately elevated glucagon secretion, slowing of gastric emptying, and reduction of food intake."[8] As you can tell by the vernacular, the American Pharmacists Association was involved in this one. So, maybe this li'l old fat lady's solution of just avoiding PSS rich foods is not so insane after all.

OK, back to the numbers. Colorado has the highest mean elevation (6,800 feet) of any state as well as the highest low point (3,317 feet). California's mean elevation (2,900 feet) is actually lower than Colorado's lowest point, and California's low point (-282 feet) is *really* low. Now, let's look at the two most obese states in the country. Alabama's mean altitude is 500 feet and Mississippi's mean altitude is 300 feet.[9] So my logic predicts that, when you factor in high altitude with high natural amenities, Colorado will win the obesity game every time. And new medical research says I'm right!

The scientific folks are now saying they've identified a strong association between obesity prevalence and altitude in the US. They're saying there's a huge 4-5 fold increase in obesity prevalence at low altitudes. And they're finding that high altitude doesn't just result in lower obesity rates. The medical researchers are also now saying that people living at higher altitudes have a lower chance of dying from ischemic heart disease and tend to live longer than others. For all the details and reference sources, check out my Author Update information on pages 259-260.

Now I want to stress a point here. As an extremely obese person, I lived in Lake County, Colorado, for approximately two years before I began to lose weight. When I moved here my weight stabilized, but I didn't actually lose weight. It wasn't until I got fed up and began eating low PSS foods that my weight began to dramatically drop. So my logic says that high altitude may help us lose weight and keep it off, but a low PSS diet is the essential component to regain our personal freedom and health.

Now, we can't all live at 10,000 feet in Colorado, so what's the point? The point is, understanding why the numbers are the way they are can help both businesses and individuals devise strategies to improve their situations and balance sheets. For example, if I am a physical exercise business owner who wants to capture the future physical entertainment market, it would make sense for me to target markets partially based upon low natural amenities. Why? Because that's where folks are desperate for physical entertainment options.

The opposite holds true for other business owners. With the American economy struggling to remain viable, businesses are desperately seeking ways to control costs. In decades past, businesses focused on locating the majority of their functions where there was a favorable business/tax environment and a good pool of qualified labor. This li'l old fat lady believes it is possible that future decisions on where to locate new business ventures may also factor in geographic areas where lower obesity rates exist. With the average adult overweight and obesity rate in America now at 68.5% and still rising, a nice, lean, healthy labor pool could become increasingly rare as time goes on. This may sound a little far-fetched but, just a few decades ago, many folks didn't predict that most of our big American businesses would relocate their customer service operations to places like the Philippines.

At the current time, as health care costs continue to escalate out of control, more and more businesses are beginning to pass those escalating costs on to their employees. And they are penalizing the obese and smokers by making them pay more. Here's what a 2011 Reuters Health Information article says.

> Overall, the proportion of large and midsized companies using penalties is expected to climb in 2012 to almost 40%, up from 19% this year and only 8% in 2009, according to an October survey by consulting firm Towers Watson and the National Business Group on Health. The penalties include higher premiums and deductibles for individuals who failed to participate in health management activities as well as those who engaged in risky health behaviors such as smoking.
>
> The weak economy is contributing to the change. Employers face higher health care costs in part because they're hiring fewer younger healthy workers and losing fewer more sickly senior employees.
>
> The poor job market also means employers don't have to be as generous with these benefits to compete. They now expect workers to contribute to the solution just as they would to a 401(k) retirement plan, says Jim Winkler, a managing principal at consulting firm Aon Hewitt's health and benefits practice. "You're going to face consequences based on whether you've achieved or not," he says.
>
> And those that don't are more likely to be punished. An Aon Hewitt survey released in June (2011) found that almost half of employers expect by 2016 to have programs that penalize workers "for not achieving specific health outcomes" such as lowering their weight, up from 10% in 2011.
>
> These changes come at a time when health insurance premiums are soaring. In 2011, the average cost of an employer-provided family plan was more than $15,000, according to a survey by the Kaiser Family

Foundation and the Health Research and Educational Trust. That's 31% higher than five years ago. And the number is expected to climb another 5% to 8% next year, according to various estimates.

And there are also those that no matter how much they exercise or how healthy they eat can't lose weight or lower their blood pressure or body mass index. "There are thousands and thousands of people whose paycheck is being cut because of factors beyond their control," says [Lewis] Maltby from the National Workrights Institute."[13]

In response to Lewis Maltby's statement, *"There are thousands and thousands of people whose paycheck is being cut because of factors beyond their control,"* as a li'l old fat lady who's been there, done that, I say *nonsense!* Show me a single example of an overweight or obese person who has a Big Mac in his or her hand and a gun pointed to his or her head. Yes, today you must defy current diet doctrine to regain your personal freedom and health. But the person responsible for your current situation is you. If I can get fed up, lose 90 pounds, and regain my health and personal freedom without dieting, you can, too.

But, right now, you must defy current diet doctrine to be successful. A little later in this book, you will read about "Foods and Recipes That Will Knock Your Socks and 90 Pounds Off" in chapter 9. You don't need to diet and be hungry, but you do need to make sure you are only eating low PSS foods. If you follow this simple rule, you *can* permanently lose excess weight and regain your personal freedom and health. You can also avoid being punished by your employer with higher health care costs.

If you're a business owner, you can either continue down the slippery path of passing your escalating health care costs on to your employees or try to find some other way to change the game. Until Americans 'fess up and begin eating more low PSS foods, the only way to change the game is to locate your business where the healthy, slim folks are. States and counties who have smart economic development corporation staffs may be able to seize this opportunity to attract new businesses. A nice, lean, healthy labor pool may eventually become a bigger economic draw to prospective businesses than a favorable business/tax environment!

Looking at geography is not just limited to the big corporations. The same thing holds true for the obese individual. When you realize that you live in a place where natural amenities are lacking and obesity rates are high, you can either move or think about finding other ways to engage in physical entertainment. If you live in a cold, damp or hot, damp climate, maybe seeking some indoor activity that makes you physically move would be worth considering. It doesn't have to be extremely hard or challenging. The trick is to find *anything* pleasurable that will get you to move a little each and every day. We're not talking exercise here, but simply moving.

Here's an example, even though it doesn't always involve pleasure. There's an interesting anomaly in the low obesity rates for the top 50 counties. California's San Francisco County, with a black and Hispanic population of 21.7%, is listed in the top 50 with an obesity rate of 17.2% and a natural amenity ranking of six (high) out of 3,111. However, New York County, with a black and Hispanic population of 44.1%, beats San Francisco County with a 15.2% obesity rate, but it has a natural amenity ranking of 1,684 (low) out of 3,111. Judging by natural amenities and minorities, New Yorkers should be much fatter than San Franciscans. So what's going on?

This li'l old fat lady's explanation is that most New Yorkers don't climb into their cars to go to work and go shopping. Nope, New York's massive public transportation systems require most folks to walk a little every day, even if it's not always for pleasure. Driving and parking a car in downtown New York is not for the timid or poor. So even this low level of daily physical activity probably makes a big difference over the long haul.

Now, I've got another interesting observation. Turns out that the counties with the very lowest natural amenity ratings don't have the highest obesity rates. Here's a list of the ten lowest ranked natural amenity counties in the country along with their stats.

BOTTOM 10 COUNTIES RANKED BY *NATURAL AMENITY*
(Low Amenity Ranking = High Number)

STATE	COUNTY	AMENITY RANKING	% OBESITY	% DIABETES	% INACTIVE
MN	PENNINGTON	3102	28.1	8.6	23.1
ND	GRAND FORKS	3103	30.9	7.4	23
MN	DODGE	3104	31.3	7.2	19.6

ND	TRAILL	3105	32.6	6.3	29.8
MN	MOWER	3106	28.5	7.2	21.8
ND	PEMBINA	3107	32.7	8	29.7
MN	NORMAN	3108	30.4	8.1	21.2
IN	TIPTON	3109	30.4	9.3	28.2
MN	WILKIN	3110	28.6	7.2	25
MN	RED LAKE	3111	31.8	7.2	19.8
	AVERAGE BOTTOM	**3106**	**30.5**	**7.7**	**24.1**

Does anybody besides me see that the list is dominated by Minnesota and North Dakota? While the obesity, diabetes, and physical activity rates are not wonderful, they're definitely not the worst in the country. Let's compare these stats with Green County, Alabama, which has the highest obesity rate in the country.

	AMENITY RANKING	% OBESITY	% DIABETES	% INACTIVE
Bottom 10 Counties	3,106 (low)	30.5%	7.7%	24.1%
Green County, AL	1,472 (high)	47.9%	16.2%	37.3%

So what's going on? Just maybe cold-weather climates have a lower obesity rate than warm -weather climates? Why might that be? I live at 10,000 feet and the weather can get a little cold and snowy during the winter months. When I'm out in subzero temperatures shoveling snow at high altitude, I can't believe that my body doesn't need just a little more low PSS food. Even though Minnesota and North Dakota don't have the altitude of Colorado, they sure do have the cold weather climate and snowy conditions. So, maybe there's something going on here, too. I bet the statisticians and scientists can't prove me wrong on this one either. Are there any takers?

With the new data coming in from the 2010 census, various news media outlets have been offering their insights. Here's one from CNN: "But the best news might be for older males." CNN quotes Carrie Werner, a statistician at the Census Bureau. "Males show more rapid growth in the older population than females over the decade. While females continue to outnumber males in the older ages, males continued to close the gap over the decade by increasing at a faster rate than females." CNN continues, "The 2000 Census showed that there were just over 88 men to every 100 women age 65 and older. In 2010, there were just over 90 men to every 100 women in that age group."[14]

Now, here's another CNN report. The title is "Smoking, Obesity Slash American Life Expectancy." The article's data come from the Institute for Health Metrics and Evaluation at the University of Washington in Seattle [in a June 15, 2011, study titled, *Falling behind: life expectancy in US counties from 2000 to 2007 in an international context*]. "The most discouraging part of the report seems to be for women. Study authors found that since 1997, women's life expectancy has slipped or failed to rise in more than 850 counties. For men, it was 84 counties."[15]

Unlike the first CNN article, which thinks the news might be good for males, I think the second CNN article is more on track. I don't believe that older males are doing better, but that older females are doing worse. Here's why. For each age category from age 20 through age 59, females have a higher obesity rate than males. Then, at age 60 plus, the tables turn and there are more obese males. Why? This li'l old fat lady believes it's because the effects of 40 years of higher obesity rates are killing off the older obese women more quickly than the older obese men. Here are the numbers.[16]

Age Category	% Obese Men	% Obese Women
20–39	27.5%	34.0%
40–59	34.3%	38.2%
60-Plus	37.1%	33.6%

There is also a big correlation between life expectancy and high amenity ranking, obesity rate, diabetes rate, and inactivity. This data is from the same June 15, 2011, Institute of Health Metrics And Evaluation at the University of Washington in Seattle study titled, *Falling behind: life expectancy in US counties from 2000 to 2007 in an international context.*[17] With the exception of Alaska, I was able to match up life expectancy with amenity ranking, obesity rate, diabetes rate, and inactivity. Below are the five best and five worst counties for men and women regarding life expectancies along with their natural amenity rating, and obesity, diabetes, and physical inactivity rates.

While there are a couple of anomalies regarding natural amenity rating, the correlation between the other variables is stunning. On average, men live 14.6 years longer and women live 10.9 years longer in counties with higher natural amenities. Their obesity, diabetes, and physical inactivity rates explain why. And if we figured out what is going on in Montgomery, Maryland, and Fairfax, Virginia, maybe we could use that information to help other low amenity counties. As an aside, Marin County, California, and Montgomery, Maryland, are listed as counties having long life expectancies for both men and women.

BEST Counties for **MEN**	Age	Amenity Rating	Obesity Rate	Diabetes Rate	Inactivity Rate
VA, Fairfax	81.1	2288	23.2%	8.1%	18.7%
CA, Marin	80.8	18	15%	5.4%	12.1%
MD, Montgomery	80.7	1862	18.1%	6.5%	16.6%
CA, Santa Clara	80.6	64	21.1%	7.4%	16.6%
CO, Douglas	80.3	104	15.7%	4.6%	11.1%
AVERAGE	**80.7**	**867 (high)**	**18.6%**	**6.4%**	**15%**

WORST Counties for **MEN**	Age	Amenity Rating	Obesity Rate	Diabetes Rate	Inactivity Rate
MS, Holmes	65.9	2085	40.8%	14.1%	35.3%
MS, Quitman	66	2576	40.1%	15.1%	34.8%
MS, Tunica	66	1758	40.2%	14.2%	39.1%
WV, McDowell	66.3	2541	32.6%	14.2%	42.1%
MS, Humphreys	66.5	2227	41.4%	13.6%	33.4%
AVERAGE	**66.1**	**2237 (low)**	**39%**	**14.2%**	**36.9%**

BEST Counties for WOMEN	Age	Amenity Rating	Obesity Rate	Diabetes Rate	Inactivity Rate
FL, Collier	86	120	22.1%	7.2%	16.2%
WY, Teton	84.7	87	13.8%	4.4%	10.6%
CA, San Mateo	84.5	17	19.8%	6.5%	16.1%
CA, Marin	84.5	18	15%	5.4%	12.1%
MD, Montgomery	84.5	1862	18.1%	6.5%	16.6%
AVERAGE	**84.8**	**421 (high)**	**17.8%**	**6%**	**14.3%**

WORST Counties for WOMEN	Age	Amenity Rating	Obesity Rate	Diabetes Rate	Inactivity Rate
MS, Holmes	73.5	2085	40.8%	14.1%	35.3%
MS, Sunflower	73.6	2365	41.4%	14.4%	34.6%
MS, Humphreys	74.1	2227	41.4%	13.6%	33.4%
MS, Quitman	74.1	2576	40.1%	15.1%	34.8%
MS, Tunica	74.1	1758	40.2%	14.2%	39.1%
AVERAGE	**73.9**	**2202 (low)**	**40.8%**	**14.3%**	**35.4%**

Finally, rural counties that rank high in natural amenities with low obesity rates currently have a growing opportunity to improve their financial situation. With our urban-centric economy, many of the higher paying jobs are located only in the big cities. However, the exploding baby boomer market presents a unique opportunity for those rural counties that rate highly in the area of natural amenities and low obesity rates. In marketing vernacular, these are called factor conditions, and smart marketing can make a big difference.

Here's an example of an obvious factor condition. The entire western border of Washington State meets up with the Pacific Ocean. That's a factor condition. So, Washington State has huge industries that require the ocean. Things like shipping, seafood, sea tourism, etc. A state like Arizona doesn't have industries associated with the sea because it doesn't have this factor condition. If rural counties that rate highly in the factor condition areas of natural amenities and low obesity rates aggressively market to the exploding baby boomer market, they can see their financial situations improve dramatically.

Why? Because many retired baby boomers don't need high-paying career jobs. Those rural counties that are smart enough to market their favorable factor conditions of high natural amenities and low obesity rates to baby boomers can create a positive cash flow because every 100 retirees will create 55 jobs. For all the details and research, see pages 259-260.

Now, I realize that the mortgage and financial industry debacles have a created a mess for honest Americans who pay their mortgages. This has resulted in many baby boomers being stuck in their existing homes. According to a March 2011 report from Harvard University's Joint Center for Housing Studies, "Many seniors who planned to retire and move to a different home deferred that decision after the recent financial crisis took a toll on both the equity in their homes and their retirement accounts." According to this same report, between 2005 and 2009, the mobility rate of age 55-plus homeowners fell the most with the housing downturn with a 37.5% decline in mobility. Homeowners under age 25 suffered only a 20.6% decline in mobility.[18]

I've been told that HUD (Housing and Urban Development) and USDA Rural Development have major turf battles and fight with each other, but just maybe the 78-million-plus baby boomers could persuade HUD and USDA Rural Development to offer baby boomers some relief. Both of these government agencies offer housing programs for deserving individuals. HUD is urban and USDA is rural. Maybe HUD could take over existing urban houses if baby boomers purchased rural houses through USDA

Rural Development? Yes, I know urban folks will scream foul play, but HUD could actually stimulate the urban housing market if they would just offer some innovative new programs.

USDA Rural Development already offers a "Guaranteed Loan" program for moderate income folks that sort of says they'll "co-sign" the loan. Since our financial institutions have turned into giant turtles, they love the USDA Guaranteed Loan program because they'll get paid if the borrower goes belly up. This way the financial institutions get to make money without incurring any risk and the USDA isn't out any money unless there's a problem. If HUD and USDA Rural Development won't step up to the plate, there are Fannie Mae, Ginnie Mae, Freddie Mac, FHA, and VA. Since all of these agencies are sponsored by the federal government, it would be really refreshing to see one or more of them step up to the plate and offer senior citizens and everyone else some real value. So, AARP (American Association of Retired Persons)—hello! Maybe you could help us 78-million-plus baby boomers put some pressure on Washington?

If we go down the USDA Rural Development/HUD path, we just need to demand certain levels of performance from these agencies. I would like to offer up the wise advice that my beloved banker gave me when I built three homes for low-income first-time home buyers in Leadville, Colorado. It was that most builders are not willing to suffer the brain damage (banker's words) of dealing with the USDA Rural Development folks. Unfortunately, I discovered that he was right. As the builder, I was subjected to all sorts of ridiculous things, including being required to have a geologist analyze foundation soil samples *after* the homeowners were living in their homes. The rest of the stuff was much worse. But, years later, I still experience pleasure at seeing signs of families thriving in the homes I built.

So, why in the world would baby boomers flock to the country instead of staying in the city? Because baby boomers who are watching themselves become obese, sick, and old will find the lure of personal freedom and health irresistible. Unlike the big cities with their physical exercise "sweat shops," rural counties with lots of natural amenities have all sorts of places where baby boomers can play. I can tell you from personal experience that "old" people over 60 years old who live in Lake County (Colorado) and the neighboring rural counties of Summit, Eagle, and Chaffee are the youngest oldsters I've ever met. None of us can stop the clock, but being normal weight and healthy makes the journey through old age a whole lot more fun. You also end up with a lot more disposable income.

And why in the world would anyone want baby boomers to flock to the country and become normal weight and healthy? Because the exploding obese sick baby boomer population is going to become a major financial detriment to the rest of America. It's already starting to happen. The chiseling of Medicare benefits are already an ugly reality. If you don't believe this li'l old fat lady, here are some recent headlines: *Medicare costs to reduce Social Security increase*[19] and *Medicare back on the brink over cuts to doctors.*[20]

Let's pause here for a moment and take a closer look. On Friday, January 14, 1977, Senator George McGovern announced the publication of the first *Dietary Goals for the United States.* That was 35 years ago. So, for 35 years, our federal government has been telling Americans to eat a diet that will make us obese and sick. It can take decades for the *real* bad boy on the block to rear his ugly head. So, now that the 20- to 30-year-olds in 1977 have become 55- to 65-year-olds in 2012 and are beginning to succumb to the effects of this scientifically unsound nutritional strategy, our federal government responds by cutting Medicare payments to doctors and increasing the cost for Medicare insurance premiums for the old folks.

This is not a new situation. "Despite competition and choice in the private insurance system, Medicare spending has grown more slowly than private insurance premiums for comparable coverage for more than 30 years. From 1970 to 2009, Medicare spending per beneficiary grew by an average of 1% less each year than comparable private insurance premiums."[21]

Then there's the Sustainable Growth Rate. "The SGR is the annual growth rate used to determine physician payments under Medicare. For 11 straight years, Congress has had to issue a temporary SGR fix to prevent massive Medicare cuts to physicians. Last year, Congress averted a 27.4% Medicare payment cut to physicians in the Middle Class Tax Relief and Job Creation Act of 2012."[22] And it's not over. On May 9, 2012, US Representatives Allyson Schwartz and Joe Heck released the Medicare Physician Payment Innovation Act of 2012—a bill that would permanently repeal the sustainable growth rate formula within the Medicare physician fee schedule. If this measure were to get approved, where does the $300 billion cost associated with a SGR repeal come from? Savings from the reduction in military operations in Iraq and Afghanistan.[23] No, it's not over.

The financial and medical care consequences are very bad news for baby boomers. Unless all doctors and medical facilities are forced to provide equal care to folks on Medicare and Medicaid, some of them won't. Medical Group Management Association (MGMA) research indicates that:

- 67.2% of medical practices are likely to limit the number of new Medicare patients unless Congress halts the cuts to Medicare reimbursement.
- 49.5% say they will stop seeing new Medicare patients.
- 27.5% indicate that they will cease treating all Medicare patients.[24]

Here's an example provided by the *Wall Street Journal*. "Mayo [Clinic]…will no longer accept Medicare patients at one of its primary care clinics in Arizona. Mayo said the decision is part of a two-year pilot program to determine if it should also drop Medicare patients at other facilities in Arizona, Florida, and Minnesota, which serve more than 500,000 seniors. Mayo says it lost $840 million last year [2009] treating Medicare patients, the result of the program's low reimbursement rates. Its hospital and four clinics in Arizona…lost $120 million. Providers like Mayo swallow some of these Medicare losses, while also shifting the cost by charging more to private patients and insurers… Mayo is probably a leading indicator of where other hospitals and doctors are headed. Physicians on average earn 20% to 30% less from Medicare than they do from private patients, and many are dropping out of the program."[25]

Unfortunately, as many seniors are discovering, Medicare coverage does not guarantee medical care access. Let me give you a real life example. A few years ago, a Colorado Medicare patient needed a minor "transtracheal oxygen" procedure done because she suffered from dementia and would remove her nasal cannula, thus depriving herself of oxygen. At times, her pulse oxygen would end up being in the mid 60% range whereas 95%-100% is considered normal.[26] Medicare's standard is 88%. It is below this point that damage to the heart may result.

The Denver, Colorado, metropolitan area has a population of almost 2.5 million[27] (includes Denver, Jefferson, Arapahoe, Adams, Douglas, and Broomfield Counties). In the case of this Medicare patient, it was almost impossible to find a "transtracheal oxygen" doctor who accepted Medicare *and* who operated at a medical facility that accepted Medicare. In the Denver, Colorado, metropolitan area of almost 2.5 million, there was only *one* doctor-medical facility combination available for this Medicare patient. If this Medicare patient carried regular health insurance, she would have had numerous health care provider options. How do I know this story is true? Because I'm the one who was trying to get this poor, sick old woman the medical care she needed. And this horrible inhumane real life example is going to become the norm for baby boomers unless America 'fesses up and decides it's time to turn our Titanic around.

So, back to why we want healthy, normal weight baby boomers. Sick, obese baby boomers are like old cars that have been poorly maintained—we break more often. But, unlike old cars, we'll require less in the way of maintenance if we become normal weight and healthy. For example, an analysis of cost data from several major national databases confirms that the cardiovascular risk factors of patients with a BMI over 35 cost healthcare payers an average of about $3,600, or over double the $1,700 for patients with a BMI between 25 and 27.[28] The NIH confirms the same thing for diabetes—the health care costs are over twice as high for a diabetic.[29] But these sobering stats are just the average.

The obese, sick baby boomer costs a whole lot more. In a study titled "The Benefits of Risk Factor Prevention in Americans Aged 51 Years and Older," the *American Journal of Public Health* calculates that every 51- or 52-year-old person who suffers from obesity, diabetes, and hypertension will spend an additional $387,732. Smoking adds another $118,946. Thus, the price tag is $506,678 or just a little over a *half a million dollars per sick obese older smoker*. Here's the *Journal* statement.

> The gain in life span from successful treatment of a person aged 51 or 52 years for obesity would be 0.85 years; for hypertension, 2.05 years; and for diabetes, 3.17 years. A 51- or 52-year-old person who quit smoking would gain 3.44 years. Despite living longer, those successfully treated for obesity, hypertension, or diabetes would have lower lifetime medical spending, exclusive of prevention costs. Smoking cessation would lead to increased lifetime spending. We used traditional valuations for a life-year to calculate that successful treatments would be worth, per capita, $198,018 (diabetes), $137,964 (hypertension), $118,946 (smoking), and $51,750 (obesity). Conclusions. Effective prevention could substantially improve the health of older Americans, and-despite increases in longevity-such benefits could be achieved with *little or no additional lifetime medical spending.*[30]

That's not all. I don't know if anyone else has noticed but, here in Colorado, Alzheimer's facilities are popping up like mushrooms. The Colorado Department of Public Health has a list of more than 100 facilities, and I'm not sure that's all of them.[31] So there's lots of money to be made from those demented folks! Here's what Gary Taubes has to say about Alzheimer's disease and cancer in his book, *Why We Get Fat.*

> As it turns out, both Alzheimer's disease and most cancers—including breast cancer and colon cancer—are associated with metabolic syndrome, obesity, and diabetes. This means that, the fatter we are, the more likely we are to get cancer and the more likely we are to become demented as we age. [Regarding Alzheimer's disease, Gary quotes David Schubert and Pamela Maher, neurobiologists at the Salk Institute for Biological Studies in Sand Diego:] "There is a cluster of risk factors for Type 2 diabetes and vascular disease that include high blood glucose, obesity, high blood pressure, increased blood (triglycerides), and insulin resistance. All of these factors, both individually and collectively, increase the risk of Alzheimer's disease."[32]

And, a January 17, 2012, Associated Press report states, "US wants effective Alzheimer's treatment by 2025." The AP reports that an estimated 5.4 million Americans already have Alzheimer's or similar dementias and, by 2050, that number is expected to jump to 13 million–16 million Americans, costing $1 trillion in medical and nursing home expenditures.[33] That doesn't count the billions of dollars in unpaid care provided by relatives and friends. It also doesn't take into account the enormous human suffering of the Alzheimer's victims or their families and friends.

Many goals are being debated for a national Alzheimer's plan. Each one listed in this same AP article involves spending huge amounts of money to cope with this tragic disease. Not one goal involves the simple, cheap solution of prevention in the first place. Eliminate the high PSS content from the American diet and this tragic disease will begin to retreat. Because it takes decades of a high PSS diet to cause Alzheimer's disease, it will take decades to slowly triumph over this American tragedy, so big business shouldn't worry. There's lots of money to be made for a long time from Alzheimer's disease.

Now, if you don't believe Gary Taubes's statement about the link between obesity and cancer, here's one from Christopher J. Keto, MD, a urological oncology postdoctoral associate at Duke University Medical Center, Durham, North Carolina. "We found that overweight men were three times more likely to have their [prostate] cancer spread. Obese men were five times more likely than normal-weight men to have their cancer spread."[34] And here's another one from the March 2009 issue of the *Archives of Surgery*: "Obesity Increases Risk for Metastases in Pancreatic Cancer." "Obesity greatly increased the risk for metastasis, as well as for recurrence and death…In a series of 285 patients who underwent potentially curative surgery, a small group of obese patients with a body mass index (BMI) of more than 35 was found to have a 12-fold higher risk for lymph node metastases and an almost double risk for cancer recurrence and death, compared with all the other patients."[35]

And while we're looking at sobering stats, the CDC now reports that 50 million US adults had arthritis in 2007–2009. While 29.6% of obese adults suffer from this crippling disease only 16.9% of normal/underweight adults suffer. The CDC says that obesity may be a special problem in arthritis; one in three obese adults reports having this crippling disease.

> Obesity is associated with incident knee osteoarthritis (OA), disease progression, disability, total joint replacement, and poor clinical outcomes after joint replacement and likely has a critical role in the increasing population burden and impact of arthritis.[36]

Add Alzheimer's disease, cancer, and arthritis to the obesity equation and I'll bet those older Americans who have spent decades being addicted to carbohydrates and nicotine can end up costing the rest of us *over $1 million each* as they age. And this financial disaster doesn't address the tragic human suffering element of this horrible reality. So, maybe this Peggy Prediction is worth repeating again.

Peggy Prediction: *We're eventually going to come to the realization that excessive carbohydrate consumption doesn't rot just teeth.*

But back to healthy, normal weight baby boomers living in the country. You may think that this rural stuff for baby boomers is just a li'l old fat lady's opinion. But it's not. According to a recent *Wall Street Journal* article related to the 2010 census, "Senior citizens have become the largest and fastest-growing segment of the U.S. population, a demographic shift that influences everything from consumer behavior to health-care costs…."[37] Add in a 1999 USDA Economic Research Service report titled "Natural Amenities Drive Rural Population Change," which states, "Average 1970–96 population change in nonmetropolitan counties was 1% among counties low on the natural amenities index and 120% among counties high on the index. Most retirement counties and recreation counties score in the top quarter of the amenities index."[38] If you're still not convinced, just take a look at the new USDA ERS chart below. Based on the 2010 Census, the population change for highly rated counties is now over 150%. So this li'l old fat lady has the government numbers behind her on this one. C'mon, rural counties blessed with high amenities, market them and they will come.

Median nonmetropolitan* county population change, 1970-2010, by level of natural amenities

Percent change

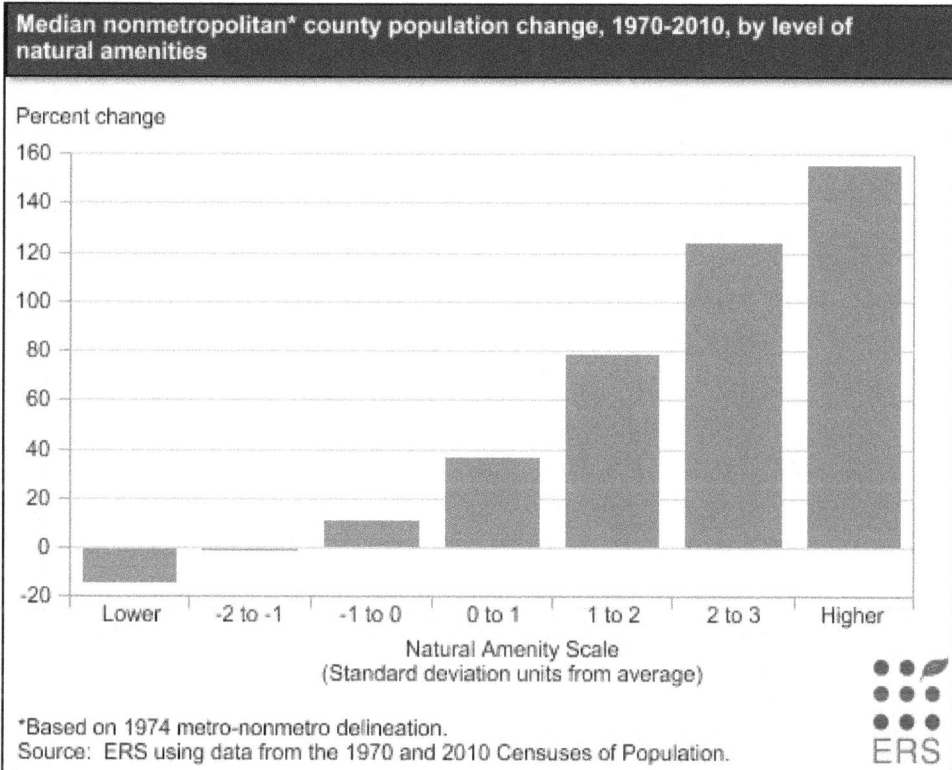

Natural Amenity Scale
(Standard deviation units from average)

*Based on 1974 metro-nonmetro delineation.
Source: ERS using data from the 1970 and 2010 Censuses of Population.

ERS 39

Now a word of caution is in order here. If folks are already suffering from nasty things including diabetes, high blood pressure, or heart disease, a lower altitude may be in order. My nearest neighbor is a registered nurse who makes a living delivering oxygen, and he tells me that high altitude can make health problems even worse. So, if you've got existing health issues, just take his expert advice into consideration. Maybe a low altitude county that is highly rated for natural amenities and has a low obesity rate might be a better option. Remember, the only essential personal freedom and health component is eating low PSS foods. Where you live is just icing on the cake.

Later on in this book, this li'l old fat lady will offer an out-of-the-box solution that would help ensure that millions of obese sick baby boomers don't financially sink America. Just maybe there *is* a way to steer our *Titanic* out of harm's way.

PART III

FOODS, RECIPES, AND PEARLS OF WISDOM

CHAPTER 8

Pearls of Wisdom

To say that the American consuming public is going to completely eliminate sweeteners out of their diet, I don't think gets us there. —Jim Simon, Board Member of the Sugar Association, Inc.

In the last seven chapters you've read about how you can join of a tiny minority of folks who lose a significant amount of weight and *keep it off*. Right now that number is less than two in 100. As a bonus, you can also become healthier. This chapter will provide you with some pearls of wisdom to help you navigate your own beautiful weight loss journey. Because I'm not a medical doctor or nutrition expert, I am generally going to refer to wisdom authored by the experts with all the right suffixes behind their names. Suffixes like MD, PhD, and RD.

But first, this li'l old fat lady strongly recommends you involve your medical doctor *before* you begin your journey. By doing so, you will increase your chances of success, and you will also have a "before" health snapshot to compare with your "after" health snapshot. It is impossible for me to describe the elation you will experience when you compare your newest lab tests with the previous ones. For me, watching diabetes and heart disease scurry away in defeat was a very joyful experience. I still smile whenever I think about how much my health has improved since I began my own weight loss journey.

But not all medical professionals have figured out that the earth is not at the center of the universe. So, how do you locate someone who can help you? Jimmy Moore's website (www.livinlavidalowcarb.com—click on Links) has a growing list of medical experts in nearly all 50 states who know how to use a healthy low-carb nutritional approach. If a physician is a member of the American Society of Bariatric Physicians (www.asbp.org) *and* is a member of the Nutrition and Metabolism Society (www.nmsociety.org) *and* is on Jimmy's physician list, chances are very good you'll get the help you need. The place to start is Jimmy's list, and then just ask the physician if he or she is a member of the ASBP and the Nutrition and Metabolism Society. If he or she is on Jimmy's list, chances are pretty good you'll get a yes to both questions.

For decades the USDA has published many versions of a food pyramid that emphasizes carbohydrates. Lots of carbohydrates—six to 11 servings a day! In June 2011, the USDA replaced MyPyramid with MyPlate as the government's primary food group symbol.[1] But the most recent 2010 USDA Dietary Guidelines still emphasize a carbohydrate-rich diet. No, the USDA has not been able to raise itself above the ideas of the time.

But Jonny Bowden's *Living Low Carb* book does offer an excellent food pyramid for those of us who understand that the earth is not at the center of the universe. Instead of emphasizing a high carbohydrate diet that leads to obesity, diabetes, heart disease, and more, Jonny's dietary pyramid emphasizes protein, fat, and vegetables. Follow Jonny Bowden's Healthy Low-Carb Life Pyramid for Life and you'll be cruising down the road to success.

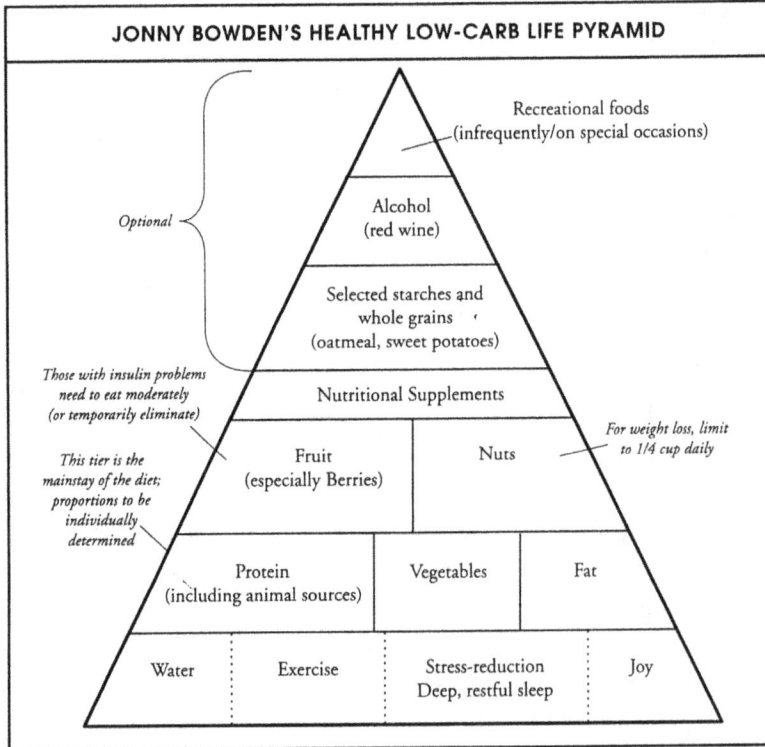

JONNY BOWDEN'S HEALTHY LOW-CARB LIFE PYRAMID

Recreational foods
(infrequently/on special occasions)

Optional

Alcohol
(red wine)

Selected starches and
whole grains
(oatmeal, sweet potatoes)

*Those with insulin problems
need to eat moderately
(or temporarily eliminate)*

Nutritional Supplements

*For weight loss, limit
to 1/4 cup daily*

*This tier is the
mainstay of the diet;
proportions to be
individually
determined*

Fruit
(especially Berries)

Nuts

Protein
(including animal sources)

Vegetables

Fat

Water | Exercise | Stress-reduction
Deep, restful sleep | Joy

OK, now that you've got the picture, let's take a look at a dietary strategy that is advocated by the Lifestyle Medicine Clinic at Duke University Medical Center.[3] In his book, *Why We Get Fat*, Gary Taubes also advocates the Duke University dietary strategy.[4] To get started, here's a little bit of history.

The driving force behind the Lifestyle Medicine Clinic's dietary strategies is a doctor named Eric C. Westman, MD, MHS. About 1998, he was a young internist in the Durham VA veteran's medical center and was in a clinical research-training program. Two of the patients he saw had lost a lot of weight and Dr. Westman asked them how they did it. Here's the story as Dr. Westman tells it.

> They said they read this little book, the Atkins Book. I said immediately, I'm going to send you to the lab because I know your cholesterol has gone up. This is how I was trained. This is where most clinicians are today, including dieticians, physicians, and nutritionists. They're going to assume the cholesterol is going up.
>
> I had a chance to check the cholesterol, and in two cases, two in a row, their cholesterol went down. There was a weight loss and a favorable change in cholesterol. So I got curious. I went to a bookstore and saw many books about low-carb diets. That Atkins one stood out, since it was the one my patients had brought in. Looking at that, I learned there was actually a clinic in operation. So I contacted Dr. Atkins, and he invited me and my staff to his clinic in New York, in 1999, and the clinic worked. The diet, I saw it in action. People were losing weight, I saw their labs; I looked over the shoulder of one of the nurses, saw the charts, and talked to people. It was really amazing to see it working. And yet what I had heard was that it couldn't work and it was unhealthy.[5]

The rest is history. Dr. Westman adopted Dr. Atkins's dietary strategies at the Lifestyle Medicine Clinic at Duke University Medical Center. He, along with Stephen D. Phinney, MD, PhD, and Jeff S. Volek, PhD, RD, are the authors of *The New Atkins for a New You* (2010). Dr. Westman is now the president elect of the American Society of Bariatric Physicians. He's also a member of the Nutrition and Metabolism Society and is on Jimmy Moore's physician list.

So, why did this li'l old fat lady pick the Duke University Medical Center dietary strategy? Well, this dietary strategy pretty much reflects what I did as I went through my 90-pound weight loss journey. But I just figured out how to have my cake and eat it too, while doing pretty much what the Duke University Medical Center experts are recommending. I'll show you how in the next chapter, "Foods and Recipes That Will Knock Your Socks and 90 Pounds Off." But first, here is the Lifestyle Medicine Clinic's dietary strategy.

Lifestyle Medicine Clinic
Duke University Medical Center

"No Sugar, No Starch" Diet: Getting Started

This diet is focused on providing your body with the nutrition it needs, while eliminating foods that your body does not require, namely, nutritionally empty carbohydrates. For most effective weight loss, you will need to keep the total number of carbohydrate grams to *fewer than 20 grams per day.* Your diet is to be made up exclusively of foods and beverages from this handout. If the food is packaged, check the label and make sure that the carbohydrate count is 1 to 2 grams or less for meat and dairy products, 5 grams or less for vegetables. All food may be cooked in a microwave oven, baked, boiled, stir-fried, sautéed, roasted, fried (with no flour, breading, or cornmeal), or grilled.

WHEN YOU ARE HUNGRY, EAT YOUR CHOICE OF THE FOLLOWING FOODS:

Meat: Beef (including hamburger and steak), pork, ham (unglazed), bacon, lamb, veal, or other meats. For processed meats (sausage, pepperoni, hot dogs), check the label. Carbohydrate count should be about 1 gram per serving.

Poultry: Chicken, turkey, duck, or other fowl.

Fish and Shellfish: Any fish, including tuna, salmon, catfish, bass, trout, shrimp, scallops, crab, and lobster.

Eggs: Whole eggs are permitted without restrictions.

You do not have to avoid the fat that comes with the above foods. You do not have to limit quantities deliberately, but you should stop eating when you feel full.

FOODS THAT MUST BE EATEN EVERY DAY:

Salad Greens: 2 cups a day. Includes arugula, bok choy, cabbage (all varieties), chard, chives, endive, greens (all varieties, including beet, collards, mustard, and turnip), kale, lettuce (all varieties), parsley, spinach, radicchio, radishes, scallions, and watercress. (If it is a leaf, you may eat it.)

Vegetables: 1 cup (measured uncooked) a day. Includes artichokes, asparagus, broccoli, Brussels sprouts, cauliflower, celery, cucumber, eggplant, green beans (string beans), jicama, leeks, mushrooms, okra, onions, peppers, pumpkin, shallots, snow peas, sprouts (bean and alfalfa) sugar snap peas, summer squash, tomatoes, rhubarb, wax beans, zucchini.

Bouillon: 2 cups daily–as needed for sodium replenishment. Clear broth (consommé) is strongly recommended, unless you are on a sodium-restricted diet for hypertension that is recommended by your doctor.

FOODS ALLOWED IN LIMITED QUANTITIES:

Cheese: Up to 4 ounces a day. Includes hard, aged cheeses such as Swiss and Cheddar, as well as Brie, Camembert blue, mozzarella, Gruyere, cream cheese, goat cheeses. Avoid processed cheeses, such as Velveeta. Check the label; carbohydrate count should be less than 1 gram per serving.

Cream: Up to 2 tablespoonfuls a day. Includes heavy, light, or sour cream (not half and half).

Mayonnaise: Up to 2 tablespoons a day. Duke's and Hellmann's are low carb. Check the labels of other brands.

Olives (Black or Green): Up to 6 a day.

Avocado: up to 1/2 of a fruit a day.

Lemon/Lime Juice: Up to 4 teaspoonfuls a day.

Soy Sauces: Up to 4 tablespoons a day. Kikkoman is a low carb brand. Check the labels of other brands.

Pickles, Dill or Sugar-Free: Up to 2 servings a day. Mt. Olive makes sugar-free pickles. Check the labels for carbohydrates and serving size.

Snacks: Pork rinds/skins; pepperoni slices; ham, beef, turkey, and other meat roll-ups; deviled eggs.

THE PRIMARY RESTRICTION: CARBOHYDRATES

On this diet, no sugars (simple carbohydrates) and no starches (complex carbohydrates) are eaten. The only carbohydrates encouraged are the nutritionally dense, fiber-rich vegetables.

Sugars are simple carbohydrates. *Avoid these kinds of foods:* white sugar, brown sugar, honey, maple syrup, molasses, corn syrup, beer (contains barley malt), milk (contains lactose), flavored yogurts, fruit juice, and fruit.

Starches are complex carbohydrates. *Avoid these kinds of foods:* grains (even "whole" grains), rice, cereals, flour, cornstarch, breads, pastas, muffins, bagels, crackers, and "starchy" vegetables such as slow-cooked beans (pinto, lima, black beans), carrots, parsnips, corn, peas, potatoes, french fries, potato chips, etc.

FATS AND OILS

All fats and oils, even butter, are allowed. Olive oil and peanut oil are especially healthy oils and are encouraged in cooking. Avoid margarine and other hydrogenated oils that contain trans fats.

For salad dressings, the ideal dressing is a homemade oil-and-vinegar dressing, with lemon juice and spices as needed. Blue-cheese, ranch, Caesar, and Italian are also acceptable if the label says 1 to 2 grams of carbohydrate per serving or less. Avoid "lite" dressings, because these commonly have more carbohydrate. Chopped eggs, bacon, and/or grated cheese may also be included in salads.

Fats, in general, are important to include, because they taste good and make you feel full. You are therefore permitted the fat or skin that is served with the meat or poultry that you eat, as long as there is no breading on the skin. *Do not attempt to follow a low-fat diet!*

SWEETENERS AND DESSERTS

If you feel the need to eat or drink something sweet, you should select the most sensible alternative sweetener(s) available. Available alternative sweeteners are: Splenda (sucralose), NutraSweet (aspartame), Truvia (stevia/erythritol blend), and Sweet'N Low (saccharin). Avoid food with sugar alcohols (such as sorbitol and maltitol) for now, because they occasionally cause stomach upset, although they may be permitted in limited quantities in the future.

BEVERAGES

Drink as much as you would like of the allowed beverages; do not force fluids beyond your capacity. The best beverage is water. Essence-flavored seltzers (zero carbs) and bottled spring and mineral waters are also good choices.

Caffeinated beverages: Some patients find that their caffeine intake interferes with their weight loss and blood sugar control. With this in mind, you may have up to 3 servings of coffee (black, or with artificial sweetener and/or cream), tea (unsweetened or artificially sweetened), or caffeinated diet soda per day.

ALCOHOL

At first, we ask that you avoid alcohol consumption on this diet. At a later point in time, as weight loss and dietary patterns become well established, alcohol in moderate quantities, if low in carbohydrates, may be added back into the diet.

QUANTITIES

Eat when you are hungry; stop when you are full. The diet works best on a "demand feeding" basis—that is, eat whenever you are hungry; try not to eat more than what will satisfy you. Learn to listen to your body. A low-carbohydrate diet has a natural appetite-reduction effect to ease you into the consumption of smaller and smaller quantities comfortably. Therefore, do not eat everything on your plate just because it's there. On the other hand, don't go hungry! You are not counting calories. Enjoy losing weight comfortably, without hunger or cravings.

It is recommended that you start your day with a nutritious low-carbohydrate meal. Note that many medications and nutritional supplements need to be taken with food at each meal, or three times per day.

IMPORTANT TIPS AND REMINDERS

The following items are *not* on the diet: sugar, bread, cereal, flour-containing items, fruits, juices, honey, whole or skimmed milk, yogurt, canned soups, dairy substitutes, ketchup, sweet condiments and relishes.

Avoid these common mistakes: Beware of "fat-free" or "lite" diet products, and foods containing "hidden" sugars and starches (such as coleslaw or sugar-free cookies and cakes). Check the labels of liquid medications, cough syrups, cough drops, and or other over-the-counter medications that may contain sugar. Avoid products that are labeled "Great for Low-Carb Diets!"

LOW-CARB MENU PLANNING

What does a low-carbohydrate menu look like? You can plan your daily menu by using the following as a guide:

Breakfast
Meat or other protein source (usually eggs).
Fat source—This may already be in your protein; for example, bacon and eggs have fat in them. But if your protein source is "lean," add some fat in the form of butter, cream (in coffee), or cheese.
Low-carbohydrate vegetable (if desired)—This can be in an omelet or a breakfast quiche.

Lunch
Meat or other protein source.
Fat source—If your protein is "lean," add some fat, in the form of butter, salad dressing, cheese, cream, or avocado.
1 to 1½ cups of salad greens or cooked greens.
½ to 1 cup of vegetables.

Snack
Low-carbohydrate snack that has protein and/or fat.

Dinner
Meat or other protein source.
Fat source—If your protein is "lean," add some fat in the butter, salad dressing, cheese, cream, or avocado.
1 to 1½ cups of salad greens or cooked greens.
½ to 1 cup of vegetables.

A SAMPLE DAY MAY LOOK LIKE THIS:

Breakfast
Bacon or sausage
Eggs

Lunch
Grilled chicken on top of salad greens and other vegetables, with bacon, chopped eggs, and salad dressing

Snack
Pepperoni slices and a cheese stick

Dinner
Burger patty or steak
Green salad with other acceptable vegetables and salad dressing
Green beans with butter

READING A LOW-CARB LABEL
Start by checking the nutrition facts.

- Look at serving size, total carbohydrate, and fiber.

- Use total carbohydrate content only.

- You may subtract fiber from total carbohydrate to get the "effective or net carb count." For example, *if there are 7 grams of carbohydrate and 3 grams of fiber, the difference yields 4 grams of effective carbohydrates.* That means the effective carbohydrate count is 4 grams per serving.

- No need to worry—at this point—about calories or fat.

- Effective carbohydrate count of vegetables should be 5 grams or less.

- Effective carbohydrate count of meat or condiments should be 1 gram or less.

- Also check the ingredient list. Avoid foods that have any form of sugar or starch listed in the first 5 ingredients.

Sugar by any other name is still sugar!

All of these are forms of sugar: sucrose, dextrose, fructose, maltose, lactose, glucose, honey, agave syrup, high-fructose corn syrup, maple syrup, brown-rice syrup, molasses, evaporated cane juice, cane juice, fruit-juice concentrate, corn sweetener.[6]

That's it. You now have Dr. Westman's dietary strategy. But here's a question you may be asking. Is the Duke University Lifestyle Medicine Clinic's carbohydrate-restricted diet exactly like Dr. Atkins's diet from almost 40 years ago? This li'l old fat lady's answer is that it's very similar, with a few changes because the past four decades have taught the nutrition experts a thing or two. The most important difference I can find is that, back in 1972, *Dr. Atkins' Diet Revolution* book recommended adding back in carbohydrates about five grams at a time as you were nearing your weight loss goal. The emphasis back then was not on fat.

Although the old way of thinking involved adding back in carbohydrates a little at a time, this li'l old fat lady's pancreas is so cranky that I can't get away with adding back *any* carbohydrates. At first, I thought I was just special. But, I guess I'm not; there are many other folks out there like me. Each of us has our own carbohydrate tolerance threshold, and some of us can tolerate more carbohydrate than others. Only by working with your doctor and watching how your body responds to this dietary strategy will you discover what your carbohydrate tolerance is. It's just a process of fine tuning a very good dietary strategy.

Jeff S. Volek, PhD, RD, and Stephen D. Phinney, MD, PhD, have written a new book, *The Art and Science of Low Carbohydrate Living*. While much of what they advocate is very similar to what Dr. Atkins recommended almost forty years ago, there's one important difference. The difference is fat. Instead of adding back carbohydrates, they recommend adding back more fat. A picture is worth a thousand words so let's take a look at a couple of pictures from *The Art and Science of Low Carbohydrate Living*.[7]

Intake and Expenditure Across Four Diet Phases

Nutrient Intake Across Four Diet Phases

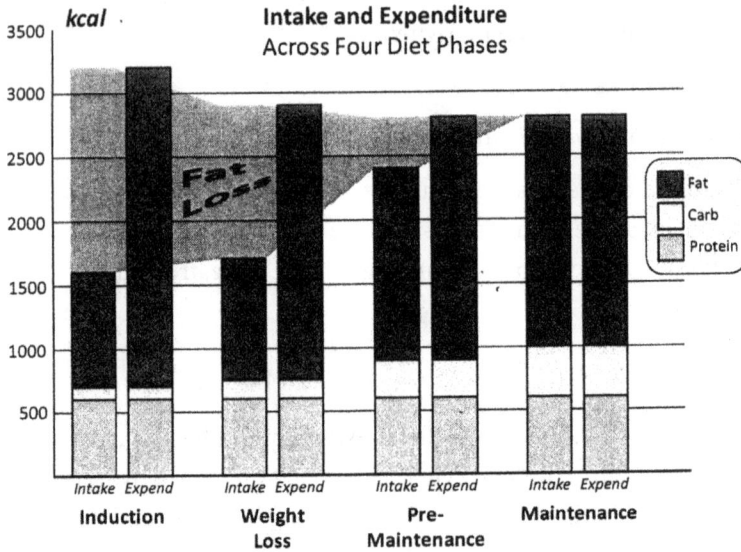

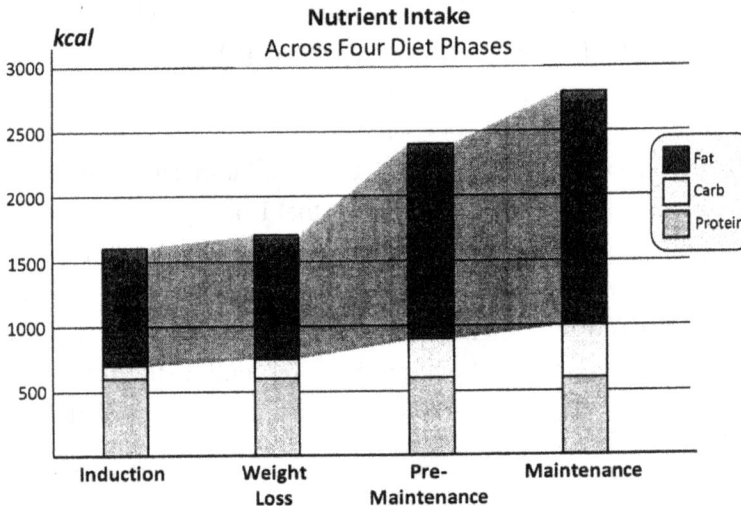

Example: Daily caloric intake and expenditure in a 5'10" man losing from 230 to 180 lbs (top) and breakdown of nutrient intake emphasizing progressive increase in fat calories (bottom). Assumes 30 kcal/kg before and 35 kcal/kg after weight loss.

See how protein intake stays pretty much the same? Carbohydrate intake stays pretty much the same too. But fat intake increases across the four diet phases recommended by *The Art and Science of Low Carbohydrate Living*. In this li'l old fat lady's opinion, these two expert authors have hit the nail right on the head. A dietary strategy that emphasizes protein and fat over carbohydrate will allow you to win your health and freedom.

But I didn't know about these two expert authors when I went through my weight loss journey. And *The Art and Science of Low Carbohydrate Living* book wasn't published until 2011. By that point, I had already gone through my 90-pound weight loss journey.

Here's what I did differently. I didn't diet at all. I just restricted carbohydrates but ate all the protein and fat I wanted from the very beginning. So, if I were to guess, I'd say I probably fell right in the middle between "Weight Loss" and "Pre-Maintenance" for the whole time. The first year I lost about 45 pounds. It took two more years to lose the remaining 45 pounds. As I got nearer and nearer to my weight loss goal, my weight loss slowed to a trickle. Sometimes it would stop for months and my weight would actually go a little in the wrong direction. But I managed to do something that less than two people in 100 do. I didn't regain all the weight I had lost and more. No, I managed to win my health and freedom.

Permanently changing the way I ate was more important to me than losing weight quickly. And by losing weight slowly, my body was able to adjust so I don't have hanging this and sagging that. But my weight loss strategies, the Duke University Lifestyle Medicine Clinic's diet strategies, and *The Art and Science of Low Carbohydrate Living*'s strategies are all very similar. All three strategies emphasize protein and fat over carbohydrates. All three strategies will allow you to win your health and freedom.

There's a new low-carb nutrition strategy term that's being adopted by many of the low-carb experts. It's LCHF, which stands for *Low Carbohydrate, High Fat*. In this li'l old fat lady's opinion, this *is* the Holy Grail. It worked for me and it can work for you. *By changing our thinking, LCHF (low carbohydrate, high fat) can turn the tide of obesity in America. Yes, it can!*

Now, here's a tip from this li'l old fat lady. Added carbohydrates lurk in almost everything we put in our mouths. Things that would normally never have sugars come with added sugars. For example, store-bought blue cheese salad dressing. It's not supposed to be the least bit sweet, but take a close look at the Nutrition Facts label. You're probably going to find a little sugar in one form or another added to this processed food. That's my point—a little sugar. All those "little sugar" additions will add up at lightening speed over the course of the day. Sort of like the numbers on the gas pump. Just one blink and you could be past Dr. Westman's recommended daily limit of 20 grams of carbs.

So here's a suggestion I'm going to make as a li'l old fat lady who's been there, done that. At the beginning of your weight loss journey, keep a small list pad with you at all times.

Every time you dump a packet of Splenda in your coffee or tea, add a "1" on the pad. Every time you put a little half-and-half in your coffee, account for it. Round up instead of down. Do this with every single thing you put in your mouth. Don't cheat and don't forget. Make sure all those "little sugar" numbers make it onto your pad.

Do this for a week. Yes, I know it's a pain and takes valuable time from your already too-busy schedule. But you will be astonished at how quickly those carb grams add up. By keeping track of every single carb you put in your mouth for a week, you will learn exactly where the potholes are. Once you know where the potholes are, they become much easier to avoid.

Here's another way of looking at this task. You no longer have to count calories. Just substitute carb counting for calorie counting for a week and you're home free. By the end of the week you'll have changed your thinking from calorie counting to carb counting. Over time you will no longer even need to count carbs because you will know which foods are carb bargains. Trust me on this one—it works.

Last but not least, *The Art and Science of Low Carbohydrate Living* has a chapter titled "Ten Clinical Pearls." I'm going to give you the CliffsNotes version here, but I suggest that reading the unabridged version is worth the purchase price of the book. Here are the Ten Clinical Pearls, CliffsNotes style.

1. **Honor the "Schwatka Imperative."** In 1979–80, Fredererick Schwatka made a 3,000-mile trek across the Canadian Arctic. His diet consisted solely of reindeer meat, and his diary says, "When first thrown wholly upon a diet of reindeer meat, it seems inadequate to properly nourish the system and there is an apparent weakness and inability to perform severe exertive, fatiguing journeys. But this soon passes in the course of two to three weeks." So, the simple imperative is to give yourself two weeks after starting a low carb diet before beginning or increasing an exercise program or resuming a physically demanding job. (This li'l old fat lady's way of putting it is that it's sort of like going cold turkey when breaking a caffeinated coffee habit. Or putting away the cigarette pack for the last time. At first, you may feel a bit lethargic or a little out of sorts because your body is addicted to excessive carbohydrates. Be patient. You're asking your body to make a big change, so just give it a little time to adjust.)

2. **It Only Appears to be High Protein.** One's protein needs are about the same across all phases of carbohydrate restriction, whether it's your first week in Induction or your second year in weight maintenance. This means that your dietary protein intake is proportionately higher at the start of the diet when weight loss is occurring than later on when weight loss has stopped.

3. **If You Can't Lose Your Fear of Fat, You Can't Do Low Carb Maintenance.** Simply put, there is no option for weight maintenance that is simultaneously low in carbohydrate and low in fat.

4. **Be Picky About Fats.** Not all fats are the same, and you need to be selective about which ones you eat for energy. We normally get plenty of omega-6 fats, but we should pay attention about getting enough omega-3 fat. Either three fish meals per week or a gram of supplemental fish oil daily will suffice. Select foods containing olive, high-oleic safflower, and canola oils. Butter and full-fat cheese are OK, and trimming fat off of meat and skin off of poultry is no longer necessary. When possible, avoid mayonnaise and dressings made with soybean, corn, sunflower, and cottonseed oils.

5. **The Salt Paradox.** When the human body adapts to a low carb diet, the kidneys fundamentally change how they handle sodium. Removing most carbs from the diet causes your kidneys to aggressively secrete sodium (and along with it, extra fluid). If you are eating less than 60 grams of carbohydrate per day, most people need to purposefully add two to three grams of sodium per day. (This is one of those areas where you may want to check in with your doctor.)

6. **Don't Trust the Bathroom Scale With Your Mental Health.** We all live inside a four-pound-wide grey zone, so that from day to day we fluctuate up or down two pounds. For people who weigh themselves frequently, this can be maddening. There are two solutions to this problem. One, just don't weigh yourself. Or two, defeat this variability by calculating average weights.

7. **Exercise is a Wellness Tool. It is Not a Weight Loss Tool.** Implement carbohydrate restriction first, lose some weight, and then decide when to become more active once you are lighter of foot. (This li'l old fat lady lost almost 20 pounds before I did much of anything.)

8. **A Sore Muscle is a Swollen Muscle.** Exercising an unfit muscle causes soreness. Don't be surprised to see the scale go up, because muscle soreness indicates that your muscles are temporarily inflamed, and inflammation causes fluid retention and swelling of the muscle.

9. **Muscle Cramps: Unnatural Complications of a Highly Refined Diet.** Muscle cramps are the end result of many contributing factors, including overuse, dehydration, and mineral inadequacies. Here's the shortcut to ending most nocturnal or postexercise muscle cramps. Take three slow-release magnesium tablets daily for 20 days.

10. **In Time, Your Habits Will Change.** When people contemplate permanently eliminating most carbohydrate-rich foods from their diet, it often seems overwhelming. However once an individual gets past the first few weeks of adaption to a low carbohydrate diet, the positive changes in one's life become positively reinforcing.[8]

Other than muscle cramps, this li'l old fat lady can personally attest to the wisdom of these Ten Clinical Pearls. When you are making fundamental changes in your life, you have to lighten up and roll with the punches. Of course, when you lighten up, it *will* be much easier to roll with the punches.

Each physician who specializes in bariatric (weight loss) medicine will have his or her own list of clinical pearls. So this li'l old fat lady suggests you listen to your doctor and do what he or she says. If your physician is a member of the American Society of Bariatric Physicians (www.asbp.org) *and* a member of the Nutrition and Metabolism Society (www.nmsociety.org) *and* is on Jimmy Moore's physician list (http://www.livinlavidalowcarb.com—click on Links), chances are very good you'll get good medical advice that will allow you to win your health and freedom.

Currently, Jimmy's list has well over 200 medical professionals who understand the LCHF (Low-Carbohydrate-High-Fat) nutrition strategy. Sadly, at the time this book went to press, Alabama and Mississippi didn't have a single medical doctor listed. These two states have 27 counties with the worst obesity rates in the whole country. For the names of the counties, just go back to chapter 7 and take a look at the list of the 50 counties with the worst obesity rates in the country. So, it would be really nice if the ill overweight and obese folks in these two states had a doctor or two that could help them win their health and freedom. Are there any Alabama or Mississippi bariatric physicians out there who understand that the earth is not at the center of the universe? If so, please get on Jimmy Moore's physician list. There are lots and lots of ill overweight and obese folks in Alabama and Mississippi who will beat a path to your door.

Now, let's move on to the next chapter, where I'll tell you about some "Foods and Recipes That Will Knock Your Socks and 90 Pounds Off." Remember the picture on the front cover of the book? Remember that strawberry shortcake with the whipped cream? This is not about dieting. This is about living.

CHAPTER 9

Foods and Recipes That Will Knock Your Socks and 90 Pounds Off

How does an ant eat an elephant? One bite at a time.—African Proverb

When I first began my weight loss journey, I was very frustrated by not being able to have my cake and eat it, too. I was forced to give up too many wonderful things that I had grown up with. So I began experimenting to find replacements for as many good high PSS foods as possible. Not worrying about calories and fats really helped, and I gradually kept adding back low PSS versions of foods until I had found really good substitutes for many of the foods I had originally eliminated.

At the current time, our food and beverage industries offer very few low PSS alternatives. The processed food folks tried to jump on the 2003 "low carb craze" bandwagon, but most consumers were just not buying it. As a result, many of the early low PSS food items gradually disappeared off the grocery store shelves. At this time, many of the ingredients I use in my low PSS cooking must be ordered off the Internet.

In the final two chapters, this li'l old fat lady will offer some marketing strategies to help Americans gain more low PSS options, but obese ill folks like me can't wait. We need to get fed up now and utilize the resources we already have. If enough of us turn our backs on the processed food and fast food industries, they'll start to listen. Remember, we're the consumers and we're in charge.

So, for the time being, you need to be willing to spend more time in the kitchen to make yourself really good meals that will also make you slim and healthy. Now, I'm not talking low fat and low calorie. No, I'm talking about stuff with lots of butter, eggs, sour cream, cheese, nuts, and many other "forbidden" ingredients. Even my physician Dr. Leder expected my cholesterol levels to get worse, but the numbers just kept getting better and better until the Lipitor (high cholesterol) medication became a thing of the past.

Here's a very important point. When I say I have my cake and eat it too, that doesn't mean carbohydrates. You can't eat what I'm eating and then go and pig out on high PSS foods. So, you need to make a decision and then stick with that decision. Either you are going to pursue a high PSS lifestyle, or you're going to pursue a low PSS lifestyle. If you try to do both, you're only going to make your current situation even worse. Michael R. Eades, MD, and Mary Dan Eades, MD, say the same thing.

> …When dietary fat and cholesterol do cause problems, it's usually *because* of the carbohydrate eaten along with them. It is true that fat is the raw material from which the body makes cholesterol, and it is also true that if you add more fat to your diet your cholesterol will increase, *but only if you continue to eat a lot of carbohydrate at the same time that you add the fat.*[1]

Now, this may be a good place to discuss a serious issue that affects both diabetics and low-carb community members who wish to follow a low PSS dietary strategy. Our goal is to consume products that don't cause our blood insulin levels to increase dramatically. Currently we attempt to achieve this goal by controlling the "net carb" counts of the foods we eat. The number of carbohydrates in the food typically correlates with blood insulin level spikes. The higher the number of carbohydrates in the food, the higher the insulin spikes.

But, at this point in time, the consumer has no way of knowing if the information on the Nutrition Facts label on the back of our processed foods is accurate. No, we don't really know the nutritional content of the foods we are eating. Today, the FDA allows a 40% variance in the carbohydrate count on the Nutrition Facts label. I'll discuss this point fully in the next chapter. And, there's an indication that some "low-carb" food manufacturers might possibly be misrepresenting their product. It's today's version of Snake Oil.

Here's a little history of the term. The phrase *snake oil* is a derogatory term used to describe quackery, the promotion of fraudulent or unproven medical practices. The expression is also applied metaphorically to any product with questionable and/or unverifiable quality or benefit.

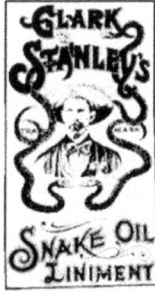

Stanley's snake oil—produced by Clark Stanley, the "Rattlesnake King"—was tested by the United States government in 1917. It was found to contain:

- mineral oil

- 1% fatty oil (presumed to be beef fat)

- red pepper

- turpentine

- camphor

The government sued the manufacturer for misbranding and misrepresenting its product, winning the judgment of $20 against Clark Stanley. Soon after the decision, "snake oil" became synonymous with false cures, and "snake oil salesmen" became a tag for charlatans.[2]

This li'l old fat lady is going to lay out the facts regarding a low carb food and let you decide whether you think you're looking at a case of modern day Snake Oil. It's the most thoroughly documented example I know of; therefore, I believe it's the best example to use. Let me stress that I am not giving you my opinion on the matter. I'm just laying out the facts.

In many grocery stores there is a product called Dreamfields. It's a pasta that claims to have *"5g Digestible Carbs Per Serving."* On the back of the box, Dreamfields states that this product has a total of 41 carbs, but 5 grams are fiber, and 31 grams are *"Protected Carbs,"* so the *"Digestible Carbs"* are 5 grams. The Nutrition Facts label just says "Total Carbohydrate 41 grams, Dietary Fiber 5 grams." That would normally mean a net carbohydrate count of 36 grams per serving.

The Dreamfields box states, *"With only 5 grams of digestible carbs, Dreamfields helps limit the rise in blood sugar levels that normally occur after eating regular pasta."* The box also states, *"Count 5 grams of carbohydrates per each 56g serving when controlling carbohydrate intake and blood sugar levels to promote good health and weight control. Dreamfields offers many health benefits and has been clinically tested to establish digestible carbohydrate levels."*[3]

How does the consumer know if these statements are true? What the heck do the terms *"Protected Carbs"* and *"Digestible Carbs"* mean? Who does the consumer contact to verify this information? How do we know we're not looking at Snake Oil? This li'l old fat lady sure doesn't know the answers.

As I said back in chapter 6, I consider Jimmy Moore to be the *Consumer Reports* of low carb. He has a wonderful website that provides all sorts of valuable information and support for the low carb community. The website is www.livinlavidalowcarb.com. I took the liberty of including some excerpts from of one of his blogs titled, *"Dreamfields President: We Stand Behind The Nutritional Claims Of Our Low-Carb Pasta."* Here is what Jimmy says.

> A scandalous controversy of sorts has risen up in the low-carb community over the past week…regarding this February 2011 *Diabetes Care* [American Diabetes Association] study that concluded the so-called "low-carb" pasta sold and marketed to people with diabetes and on low-carb diets by a company called Dreamfields Foods produces a similar blood sugar spike to traditional white pasta. If this is true, then it could be bad news for people on low-carb diets who are choosing to include Dreamfields pasta as part of their lifestyle change. So what is the real deal about this? I wanted to find out.

> On Tuesday, I contacted one of the investigators on that study named Dr. Mary C. Gannon…[who] confirmed that they did indeed conduct a study on the Dreamfields pasta because she wanted to know if it was a product she could use with her diabetic study subjects. When she inquired about the data confirming the claim that there are only 5g digestible carbohydrates in the Dreamfields pasta, Dr. Gannon told me she received no response back from the company. That's when she and her fellow low-carb researcher Dr. Frank Nuttall…decided to do this experiment comparing Dreamfields to traditional pasta.

I asked what they allowed the study participants to consume with the one 2-ounce serving of pasta and Dr. Gannon said matter-of-factly "salt and pepper only." Ewww! Pasta needs butter, cheese, and marinara sauce to taste good, but I understand the need to isolate the pasta to see what the impact it will have on blood sugar levels. The results of the first round of her study on five "old people" with average fasting blood glucose levels of 110–112 were astonishing:

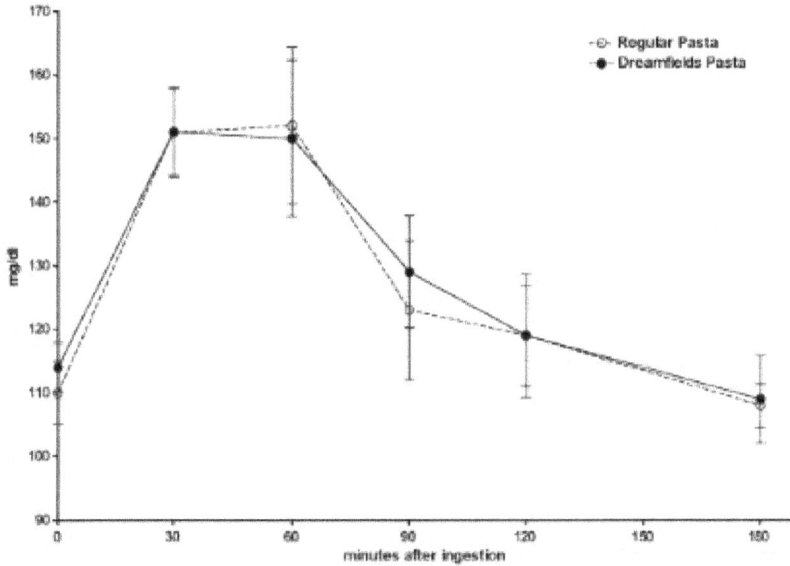

As you can see from the above graph, both the Dreamfields and traditional pasta produced similar spikes in blood sugar after consumption. Since this was an older crowd who may have had certain metabolic conditions that made their blood sugars more susceptible to this kind of response to the Dreamfields pasta, Dr. Gannon and Dr. Nuttall then decided to repeat the experiment again this time around with five "young people" with an average fasting blood glucose level of 96. Would they do any better? See for yourself:

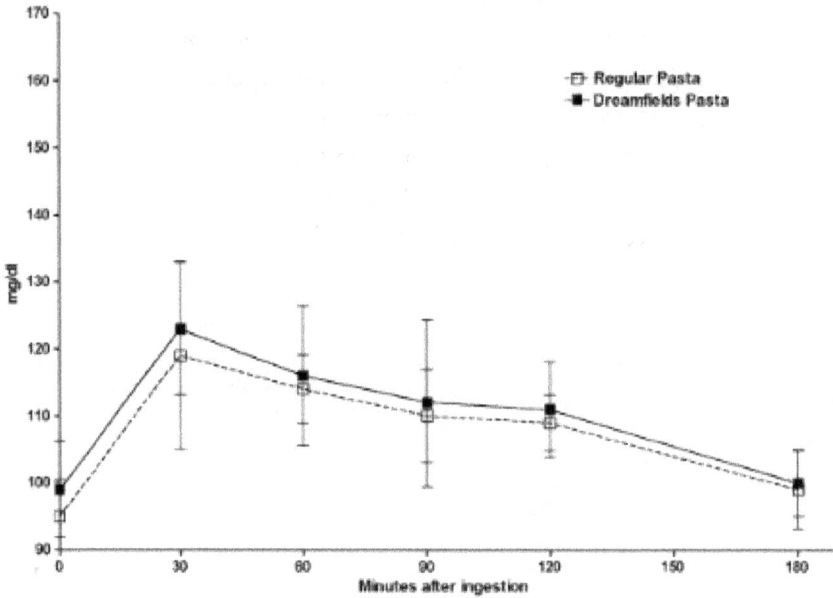

While the blood sugar rise wasn't nearly as pronounced as it was with the older study subjects, the conclusion was basically the same—the "low-carb" Dreamfields pasta produced a similar blood sugar curve as the traditional pasta. Granted, this was a very small study sample and it doesn't necessarily prove anything regarding the claims made by the Dreamfields company about their product only having 5g of what they describe as "net effective carbs."…

[The following graph is from Andreas Eenfeldt, MD], who…consumed twice the serving size (4 oz) of Dreamfields pasta in his n=1 experiment (the man is 6'7" and has more energy needs than most of us),[but] the results on his blood sugar are shocking to say the least: [The bottom line is meat, veggies, and butter. The top squiggly line is the Dreamfields.]

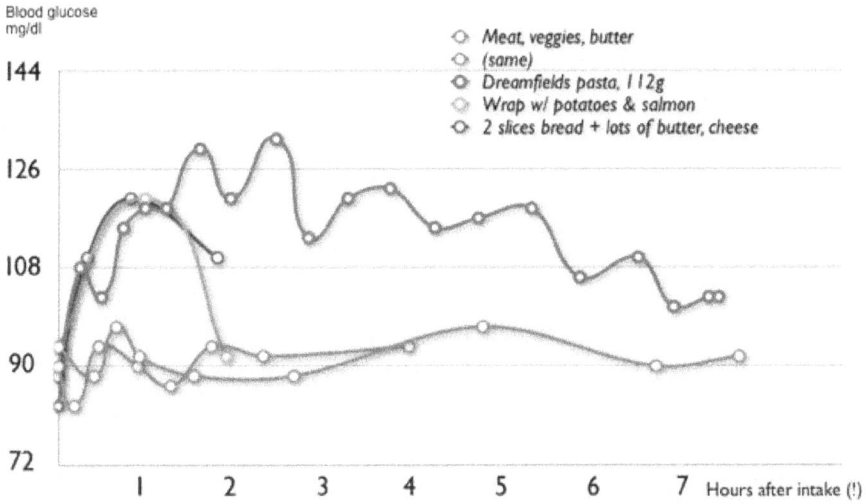

Blood glucose mg/dl

- Meat, veggies, butter
- (same)
- Dreamfields pasta, 112g
- Wrap w/ potatoes & salmon
- 2 slices bread + lots of butter, cheese

Hours after intake (!)

[Jimmy Moore then conducted a blood sugar test on himself]…In comparing the blood sugar testing results I got consuming the Dreamfields with the traditional pasta, here's what my graph looked like (special thanks to my very artistic wife Christine for drawing this for me):

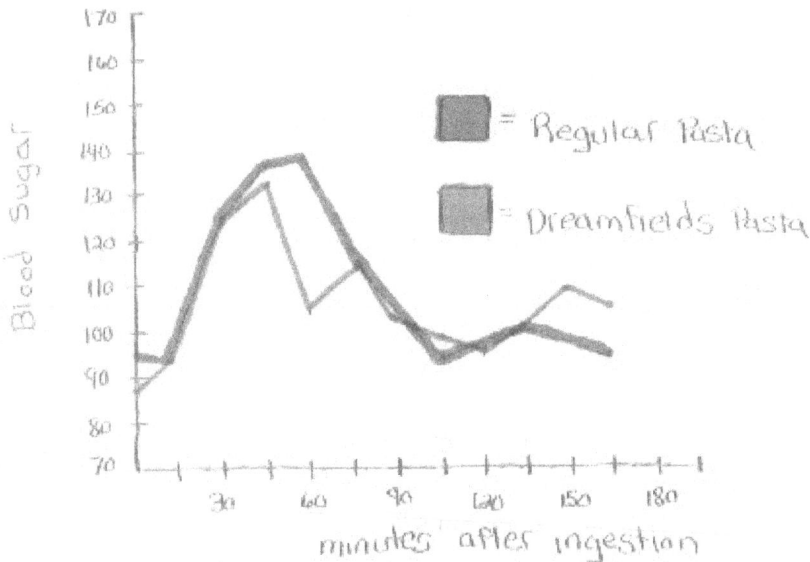

Blood Sugar

= Regular Pasta

= Dreamfields Pasta

minutes after ingestion

Needless to say, this result floored me. I suppose I was hoping the claims regarding the "protected carbs" were true, but it doesn't seem to be that way for Jimmy Moore either. The only way YOU can know how the Dreamfields pasta is going to impact you is to simply do the test for yourself...[4]

(The complete Jimmy Moore blog is located at *http://livinlavidalowcarb.com/blog/ dreamfields-president-mike-crowley-we-stand-behind-the-nutritional-claims-of-our-product/10785*).

This blog written by Jimmy Moore is a perfect example of what consumers face today when we read the packaging to evaluate the processed foods we buy. In this case, both Dr. Andreas Eenfeldt and Jimmy Moore were required to subject themselves to multiple hour, multiple needle-stick blood tests to try and determine the insulin impact of the food they were eating. This is what we consumers face today when we try to evaluate whether or not we're looking at Snake Oil.

What about the scientific study on Dreamfields conducted by the American Diabetes Association (ADA) in February 2011? Couldn't the ADA help us evaluate the insulin impact of processed foods? This is the current status of the ADA research on Dreamfields.

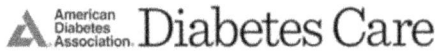

American Diabetes Association. Diabetes Care

Home | Current Issue | Archive | Contact Us | Subscribe | Help | Alert:

Withdrawn

Nuttall FQ, Gannon MC, Hoover H. Glycemic response to ingested Dreamfields pasta compared with traditional pasta. Diabetes Care 2011;34:e17–e18

This article has been withdrawn by the authors because some of the data were obtained prior to receiving IRB approval.

© 2011 by the American Diabetes Association.

[5]

Dreamfields has now agreed to a $7.9 million lawsuit settlement (see page 259-260 for details) and here's what this li'l old fat lady has to say about what you've just read. Please don't expect our government or big business to put your personal interests first. Their top priorities are to do things that will fuel the American economy and maximize next quarter's earnings. Don't expect either of them to do something that might contradict this reality.

While this may sound harsh, it's this American economic system that has made our country a powerhouse in the world for so many decades. If we want to turn the tide of obesity and ill health in America, it's up to each of us consumers to make this happen. *Yes, we do have the ability to make this happen.*

In the next two chapters, this li'l old fat lady will offer up some marketing strategies that will help eliminate the need for multiple hour, multiple needle-stick blood tests to determine the insulin impact of the foods we eat. These marketing strategies would also allow the obese ill consumers to have their cake and eat it too, while enabling many big businesses to generate nice profits for their stockholders.

Yes, there *is* a way that the obese ill consumer, big business, and big government can *all* win. But stay with me here. First, let's find out about foods and recipes that will knock your socks and 90 pounds off. After that, we'll get back around to this li'l old fat lady's marketing strategies.

As I said earlier, for the time being, you need to be willing to spend more time in the kitchen to make yourself really good meals that will also make you slim and healthy. With our wonderful Internet and Amazon.com, there's a huge array of low carb cookbooks available. One of the most prolific authors is Dana Carpender, with more than a dozen different cookbooks. Dana has also written *How I Gave Up My Low-Fat Diet and Lost 40 Pounds,*[6] and she is the managing editor of *www.CarbSmart.com*, a website that offers valuable, up-to-date information on the low-carb industry. While Dana doesn't use all the same ingredients I use, we both believe in the value of keeping your carb consumption low.

In addition to low carb cookbooks, many of the books I've already mentioned have outstanding chapters on low PSS foods and recipes. And, since they're written by medical and nutrition experts with all the right suffixes, they contain some really valuable medical advice, too. Here are the books I have.

Jeff S. Volek, PhD, RD, and Stephen D. Phinney, MD, PhD
- *The Art and Science of Low Carbohydrate Living* (2011)
- *The Art and Science of Low Carbohydrate Performance* (2012)
- *The New Atkins for a New You* (2010, along with author Eric C. Westman, MD, MHS)

Michael R. Eades, MD, and Mary Dan Eades, MD
- *Protein Power* (1999)
- *The Six-Week Cure for the Middle-Aged Middle* (2009)

Richard K. Bernstein, MD
- *Dr. Bernstein's Diabetes Solution* (2011)
- *The Diabetes Diet* (2005)

The more low PSS food alternatives you have, the better you will live. So, it's a good idea to spend a generous amount of time and effort investigating lots of resources, recipes, and ideas. In addition to providing you with low PSS recipes, I will also tell you about my favorite foods along with their current URL. URLs have a habit of changing over time, so you may need to do a search if the URL has changed.

First, here's the "OK" and "no-no" list that my physician Dr. Leder gave me so long ago. As you can see, the "no-no" list was longer and contained foods that I really loved, so I was not a happy camper. As a result, I became obsessed with keeping both the "OK" list *and* the "no-no" list. I just had to find low PSS versions of the "no-no" list foods.

"OK" LIST	"NO-NO" LIST
Animal protein, including beef, chicken, and pork	Sugar
Fish and seafood	Wheat, bread, and pasta
Hard cheeses	Corn
Eggs	Rice
Butter and fats	Potatoes
Many varieties of nuts	Beans and legumes
Dark green vegetables, including salads	Sweet vegetables, including peas and carrots
Berries	Sweet fruits
Diet sodas	Regular sodas
Decaffeinated coffee and tea	Caffeinated coffee and tea

Cream	Milk
	Sweet desserts and candy
	Alcohol

To start, let me tell you what items on the "no-no" list are still completely "no-no."

- Sugar

- Corn

- Rice

- Potatoes

- Most beans and legumes

- Sweet vegetables

- Sweet fruits

- Regular sodas

- Fully caffeinated coffee

- Most milk

- Sugar sweetened desserts and candy

- Alcohol, except once in a great while

Now, I know it looks like just about everything on the "no-no" list is still "no-no." But, read on. This li'l old fat lady has come up with a work-around for a majority of the items on the "no-no" list. And in the next two chapters, I will offer a marketing strategy that could help put many of the "no-no" list items on the "OK" list. Yes, someday we may be able to eat corn, potatoes, wheat, rice, bread, and pasta that doesn't make us sleepy, fat, and ill. But stay with me here. Let's look at where we are right now. First, I'm going to start with things you eat directly and then work my way into cooking and baking.

Since sweetness is one of the five basic taste sensations and is almost universally regarded as a pleasurable experience,[7] I'm going to begin with chocolate. Like many Americans, I'm a chocoholic and a sweetaholic. I like to eat sweets. I enjoy the taste of sweets after consuming lunch or dinner. As a matter of fact, I'm eating a few bites of delicious sugar-free dark chocolate (70% cocoa) as I type these words. I don't miss eating chocolate that is sweetened with sugar because the sugar-free chocolate tastes just as good. My addiction is the taste of sweet, not the sweetener.

Here is a sampling of the chocolates in my kitchen cabinets. The net carb count in all of them is minimal; they're generally sweetened with maltitol. When I've shared my 70% cocoa chocolate with others, many don't even realize it's not sweetened with sugar. Your biggest challenge will be finding some of these chocolates in the retail stores. Here's an example of pure frustration. Hershey makes sugar-free, dark-chocolate-covered Mauna Loa macadamia nuts. There are only 3g net carbs per 6 piece serving! Can I find them in a retail store within a 100 mile radius? Nope. Can I order them online at Mauna Loa? Nope. Can I order them from Amazon.com? Nope.[8]

BRAND	WHERE TO BUY AND MANUFACTURER URL
Valor Chocolate	Amazingly good. Many of the dark sugar-free varieties are 70% cocoa. Can't find in retail stores except rarely at TJ Maxx and Ross. Get on Valor's e-mail list and they will sometimes send out promotions. www.valorchocolate.com.
Guylian Chocolate	Great chocolate. Originally purchased at Walmart but no longer stocked. www.guylianbelgianchocolate.com.
Amberlyn Chocolate	Wonderful chocolate. Amberlyn sells only sugar-free items. Many flavor varieties. Originally found at Costco, but infrequent roadshows. Get on Amberlyn's e-mail list and they will sometimes send out promotions. www.amberlynchocolates.com.
Russell Stover, Whitman's	Bags of assorted chocolate candies. Many Walmarts and grocery stores stock. www.russellstover.com.
Hershey	Bags of sugar-free York peppermint patties, Reese's Peanut Butter Cups, etc. Many Walmarts and grocery stores stock. www.hersheyssugarfree.com.

| Dove Chocolates | Bags in many Walmarts and grocery stores. www.dovechocolate.com. |
| DeMet's Turtles | Bags in many Walmarts and grocery stores. www.demetscandy.com. |

Now let's take a look at some typically high-carb "no-no" items that the manufacturers are claiming to be low PSS products. The carb counts listed are net carbs. You will not see Splenda or Stevia in the Raw on my sweetener list because the majority ingredient in both of these products is some form of "sugar in sheep's clothing." Since there are new low PSS sweeteners coming out almost every week, I suggest you keep an eye on the grocery store shelves and frequently check out the internet for your latest options.

Here's an example. Walmart has just started exclusively stocking new liquid sweeteners made by a company called Nevella. Nevella makes Sucralose To Go, Stevia To Go, and Monk Fruit To Go. There is no "sugar in sheep's clothing" listed in these Nevella sweeteners so I bought all three to check them out. My verdict? Nevella and Walmart get a gold star for offering sweeteners that are free from "sugar in sheep's clothing." The To Go sweeteners are good for sweetening beverages. I still prefer EZ-Sweetz liquid sucralose and Sensato erythritol *powder* for cooking and baking because it's much easier to convert them to "sugar" measurements for recipes.

Now I want to stress that the carb counts I show are what the manufacturer is claiming. Unlike Dr. Andreas Eenfeldt, I am not willing to poke myself with a needle and draw blood 20-plus times in seven hours to determine my insulin response to a particular food. Dr. Eenfeldt and Jimmy Moore are my heroes, but I'm just not going there.

CATEGORY	BRANDS AND OTHER INFORMATION
Barbecue sauce	Smokin' Joe Jones. Carbs = 2g per 2 T. Add 1t of Honey Tree's "honey" per 1T of BBQ sauce for a sweeter taste. Sucralose. Online only. www.smokinjoejones.com and others.
Barbecue sauce	Nature's Hollow xylitol sweetened. Carbs = 2g per 1T serving. Hickory maple and honey mustard. Online only. www.natureshollow.com and others.
Beans	Eden organic black soy beans. Some health food stores sell these black beans in the can. Carbs = 1g carbs per ½ cup serving. www.edenfoods.com.
Bread	Bagels. Carb Krunchers. Taste good, lots of varieties, and big. Carbs = 6g per bagel. Expensive. Online only. www.lindasdietdelites.com and others.
Bread	English muffins. Nature's Grain online at Sam's Club. Carbs = 9g. Must order 72 muffins online. Sam's club Item #126032.
Bread	Hamburger/hot dog buns. Sara Lee 80 Calories and Delightful 100% Whole Wheat. Carbs = 9g per hot dog bun, Carbs = 8g per hamburger bun. In grocery stores.
Bread	Sandwich bread. Sara Lee 45 Calories & Delightful 100% Whole Wheat with Honey. Carbs = 9g per 2 slices. Make sure to get "honey" version. The other Sara Lee low-carb bread varieties have more carbs. Grocery stores stock.
Bread	Tortillas. Mission Carb Balance medium soft taco. Tastes like the "leaded" white tortillas. Carbs = 6g per tortilla. Grocery stores stock.

Bread	Tortillas. Santa Fe Tortilla Company. Homestyle whole grain. Carbs = 6g per tortilla. My local Costco carries at a reasonable price.
Bread	Tortillas. La Tortilla Factory. Low carb, high fiber. Carbs = 3g per tortilla. Grocery stores stock. Drs. Eades recommend in *The Protein Power Plan* book.
Chips	Olé Mexican Foods. Fritangas/Chicharrones de Harina, plain and with chile and lime. Carbs = 1g per oz. These are very lightweight, airy, wheat-based chips. Purchased at Walmart. www.olemexicanfoods.com.
Chips	Chicharrones or pork rinds. Various brands. Carbs = 0g carb. In most stores.
Chips	Tortillas. Mission Carb Balance listed above. Fry in 2T of butter until crisp.
Coffee	Costco Kirkland Signature Roasted by Starbucks. Comes in 2lb bags for a very reasonable price. Must grind. Mix half decaf and half regular to minimize blood sugar spikes. Tastes like caffeinated coffee but with half the caffeine.
Flour	Carbquik. Tova Industries. Wheat-based biscuit and baking mix. Carbs = 6g per cup. Online only. www.netrition.com.
Flour	Carbalose flour. Tova Industries. Wheat based baking flour. Carbs = 19g per cup. Online only. www.netrition.com.
Honey	HoneyTree's Sugar Free imitation honey. Carbs = 0g. Walmart and Target stock.
Honey	Nature's Hollow xylitol sweetened. Carbs = 2g per 1T. Online only. www.natureshollow.com and others.

Ice cream	Safeway Select Watch 'n Carbs. Vanilla (3g) and Butter Pecan (4g). Full-fat, rich ice cream sweetened with Splenda. Comes in 1.5-qt. rounds. In stores.
Jam/preserves	Polaner Sugar Free with Fiber. Splenda sweetened. Carbs = 1–2g per 1T serving. Lots of flavors, including raspberry, strawberry, apricot, marmalade, blackberry. Blueberry and peach flavors are discontinued. In stores. Difficult to find flavors.
Jam/preserves	Nature's Hollow xylitol sweetened. Lots of flavors, including apricot, peach, raspberry, strawberry, blueberry, and mountain berry. Carbs = 2g per 1T serving. Online only at www.natureshollow.com and others.
Ketchup	Heinz Reduced Sugar. Sucralose sweetened. Carbs = 1g per 1T. Grocery stores.
Ketchup	Nature's Hollow xylitol sweetened. Carbs = 2g per 1T. Online only. www.natureshollow.com and others.
Milk—dairy beverage	Hood Calorie Countdown. Tastes great. Carbs = 3g white, and 4g chocolate per 8 oz. Splenda sweetened. In grocery stores. www.hoodcaloriecountdown.com.
Milk—soy	Westsoy Organic Unsweetened. 1g net carb per 8 oz. In grocery stores.
Sauce—marinara	Victoria White Linen Collection All Natural Marinara Sauce. Costco usually stocks at reasonable price. Watch Nutrition Facts label! Net carb count varies from jar to jar, 2 net carbs to 7 net carbs per ½ cup serving.
Sauce—pasta	Bella Vita. Carbs = 4g per ½ cup serving. Online only. www.netrition and others.
Sweetener*	Truvia. Erythritol and Stevia. Carbs = 0g. In grocery stores.

Sweetener	Nevella Stevia To Go liquid. Erythritol and Stevia. Only available at Walmart.
Sweetener	SweetLeaf. Stevia. Carbs = 0g. Online only. www.netrition .com and others.
Sweetener*	EZ-Sweetz liquid sucralose. Carbs = 0g. 1 drop = 2t or 1 drop=1t. Check product to verify. Only available online at www.ez-sweetz. com and others.
Sweetener	Sweetzfree liquid sucralose. Carbs = 0g. Online only. www. sweetzfree.com and others.
Sweetener	Fiberfit liquid sucralose. Carbs = 0g. Online only. www.fiberfit.com and others.
Sweetener	Nevella Sucralose To Go liquid. Less concentrated than others. Only at Walmart.
Sweetener*	Sensato. Erythritol *powder* (not crystals). Carbs = 0g. Sometimes hard to find. Used for creaming butter and frostings in place of powdered sugar. www.Sensato.com and others.
Sweetener	XyloSweet. Xylitol crystals. Carbs = 0g. Health food stores. www. xlearinc.com.
Sweetener	Nevella Monk Fruit To Go liquid. Not as sweet. Only available at Walmart.
Sweetener	Just Like Sugar. Chicory root dietary fiber. Carbs = 1g per teaspoon. Health food stores and online. www.justlikesugarinc.com and others.
Sweetener	Steel's Gourmet Nature Sweet maltitol powder. Carbs = 0g. Online only. www.steelsgourmet.com and others.

Syrup	Joseph's in both maple and clear, like Karo Syrup. Carbs = 0g. You will want to get both. Better than store brands. Online from www.josephslitecookies.com. Free shipping. (Regarding Joseph's cookies, check the carb count.)
Syrup	Nature's Hollow xylitol sweetened. Carbs = 2g per ¼ cup. Maple and raspberry. Online only. www.natureshollow.com and others.
Tartar sauce	Kraft Lemon and Herb. Carbs = less than 1g per 2T. In grocery stores.
Thickener	Pomona's Universal (100%) Pectin. Good for thickening up all sorts of foods. Jelling power is activated by calcium, not sugar. Carb count not listed. Available from some health food stores, on Amazon, and www.pomonapectin.com.
Whipped cream	Land O'Lakes Sugar-Free Whipped Heavy Cream in can. Carbs = 0g. Splenda sweetened. Call manufacturer on 1-800-878-9762 with UPC #3450063165. Will have trouble finding in stores. A few Walmarts carry it or can order it with UPC.

*These are the sweeteners I use most frequently.

Moving right along, one of the current challenges we low PSS folks have is the large number of food flavors that aren't typically low PSS. Like the flavor of a banana. So I'm going to share one of my best health and freedom "success" secrets with you. It's LorAnn Oils. According to their website, LorAnn Oils is a family-owned and -operated business that has been a manufacturer/distributor of essential oils since 1962. It was founded by O. K. Grettenberger, who was a very active and somewhat innovative pharmacist. Originally, LorAnn bottled and distributed about eight to 10 core essential oils, and distribution was limited exclusively to pharmacies. Over the years, LorAnn's flavoring line has grown substantially with both natural and artificial oils, and they currently offer oils for foods, aromatherapy and spa, and fragrances.[9]

This li'l old fat lady discovered LorAnn Oils by accident one day at a Walmart. I bought a single flavor on a whim and have since become quite a fan of the oils. LorAnn offers many different varieties, but the ones I use are called Super Strength Flavors (100),

New Natural Flavors (10), and Bakery Emulsions (11). By my count, LorAnn offers 121 flavors just in these three varieties. As I've experimented for myself and this book, I've managed to acquire 75 of the flavors! Fortunately, many of the Super Strength Flavors come in a one-dram size for about $1.40 so it's pretty inexpensive to try out all sorts of unusual flavors. LorAnn offers free shipping for a minimum order of $75 and, if you're on their e-mail list, they will occasionally send out promotional offers. Sadly, Walmart's website doesn't currently list any of the LorAnn Oils.

I've selected my 18 favorite LorAnn Oils for cooking, baking, and smoothies and will list them here. But you might want to take a peek at www.lorannoils.com just to see all the different oils. Currently, many LorAnn customers use their oils for very high PSS sweets and baked goods. I'm sure that LorAnn Oils company founder O. K. Grettenberger would be completely astonished to learn that LorAnn Oils are now also being used to add wonderful flavors to low PSS foods.

LORANN OIL	BAKING	COOKING	VANILLA SMOOTHY	CHOCOLATE SMOOTHY
Apricot Super Strength	X	X		
Banana Naturals	X	X	X	
Blackberry Super Strength	X	X	X	
Blueberry Naturals	X	X		
Butterscotch Super Strength	X	X	X	
Canadian Maple Super Strength	X	X	X	X
Cappuccino Super Strength			X	X

Creamy Carmel Naturals	X	X	X	X
Keoke Coffee Super Strength			X	X
Lemon Bakery Emulsion	X	X		
Mint Chocolate Chip Super Strength	X	X	X	X
Orange Bakery Emulsion	X	X	X	
Peach Super Strength	X	X		
Pecan Super Strength	X	X	X	X
Praline Super Strength	X	X	X	X
Raspberry Super Strength	X	X	X	X
Strawberry Naturals	X	X	X	
Toffee Naturals	X	X	X	X

With the exception of the two emulsions (four ounces), I initially ordered all of these flavors in the one-ounce size. A flavor I hesitated on was the Canadian Maple Super Strength. But this one is an absolute must. It's got the smell and flavor of molasses but without the carbs! You can use it in baked goods instead of brown sugar. Boy, I'm getting hungry just thinking about it! In the following recipes, I'll tell you how much to use.

In addition to LorAnn flavorings, I also use lots of different spices. Because there are so many wonderful spices besides the common everyday ones, it's sometimes difficult to find them in the regular grocery stores. But, don't despair. A brand called Spice Islands has come up with a means for you to buy their zillions of spices online.

Spice Islands' spices, along with several other brands, are available from a company called Diversified Distributing. The company is located in Des Moines, IA and, like LorAnn, you can buy just one little bottle at a time. The catch is that you must order a minimum of $50 to get free shipping, but there's so many spices it would be hard not to get free shipping! Here's the web site for Diversified Distributing. http://www.yourfoodstore.com/spices. php. The only ding I must give Diversified Distributing is that, as of when this book was published, there was no nutrition label information available for their products. While the single spice varieties are not generally a problem, knowing whether there is added PSS in one of the multi-ingredient mixtures is an absolute must![10]

Because so many of the food items we low PSS folks purchase are only currently available online, this li'l old fat lady thinks maybe we ought to band together and form "low PSS food ordering support groups." We could pool our online orders and take advantage of Netrition's $4.95 flat rate shipping offer for a minimum order of $100, Amazon's free shipping offer for a minimum order of $25, LorAnn's free shipping offer for a minimum order of $75, and Diversified Distributing's free shipping offer for a minimum order of $50. There are many other low PSS food companies that also have similar offers.

Now it's time for some recipes that will Knock Your Socks and 90 Pounds Off. Since there are already lots of really good low-carb cookbooks out there for the health conscious folks, I'm going to focus on the "fast food fan" types. These are the folks who would like to become part of the slim healthy crowd but just love the food that's served at the fast food joints. You know, the hamburger, pizza, and fried chicken joints. Isn't all that fast food really bad for you? It doesn't have to be bad at all. It can be really delicious and nutritious at the same time. Seriously! I'll tell you how in the next chapter.

I'm also going to focus on "guilt trip," rich, decadent desserts and calorie-laden "sinful" foods. You are going to see more butter, cream, eggs, fat, and cholesterol than you can imagine. This is how you are going to regain your health and freedom. I can say this because I've been there done that.

The intent of these recipes is to prove that you *can* have your cake and eat it too. You're not going to find any green leaf salad or low carb vegetable recipes here. Why? Because there are so many wonderful cookbooks with literally thousands of recipes that have already been written. As I said before, Dana Carpender has over a dozen cookbooks, so go on Amazon and take a look. Whatever your taste buds are hankering for, Dana's probably got what you want. The good news is that, between Dana's ingredient list and mine, I bet you can figure out how to have your cake and eat it too.

Many of the low PSS recipes I use were originally high PSS recipes. By simply substituting low PSS flours and sweeteners, you can "retrofit" many standard recipes. As a matter of fact, the wonderful Raspberry Cream Cheese Coffee Cake you'll see shortly was originally a high PSS recipe. But, I made it a low PSS recipe simply by substituting a couple of low PSS ingredients for the high PSS ingredients. If you'll get your creative juices flowing, I bet you can see the huge potential in some of your best "leaded" recipes.

You get to eat how much you want when you want. Eat *leisurely* until you are satisfied but not stuffed. Eat when you begin to feel hungry. Quit eating when you begin to feel full. Stop thinking about calories, fat, and cholesterol. Free your mind from those thoughts of the past. Those thoughts that got you where you are today. The *old* dogma!

Yes, you *can* regain your health and freedom, but you must change your thinking. You must rise above the ideas of the time. Remember what Albert Einstein said, *"The definition of insanity is doing the same thing over and over again and expecting different results."* Yes, we *can* move beyond the dietary insanity of the past 40 years. But we must change, and the first thing we must change is our thinking. Once we change our thinking, everything else will fall into place.

To kick your "thinking change" into overdrive, I'm now going to deliver on that strawberry shortcake picture on the front cover of this book. Yes! You *can* have your cake and eat it too! When you whip this unbelievable "sweet on steroids" concoction up for yourself, you'll know what I mean. But the total net carb count is only about 7.5g. This is the type of knock your socks off recipe that helped me lose 90 pounds and regain my health and freedom.

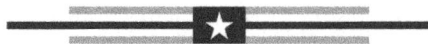

★

Peggy Tips: *After several years of experimenting with Carbquik, I finally figured out that a little squash does wonders for this product. It moistens up and improves the texture of* *your baked goods! So, don't let the squash in these recipes put you off. You won't even be able to taste it. I also use oversized muffin cups because the Carbquik dough becomes runny as it bakes and it likes to rise up quite a bit at first. Sometimes regular sized muffin cups don't quite contain the quickly rising batter and you end up with a mess on the bottom of your oven.*

You'll also notice that I use a little ground flax seed along with the Carbquik in my recipes. I think it results in a better pastry and flax seed is a good source of Omega-3 fatty acids, but you can just substitute the same amount of Carbquik, if you wish. (Costco sells large bags of organic flax seed for a very reasonable price.) If you don't want to use wheat-based flour, check out Dana Carpender's cookbooks. She uses ground almonds, whey protein powder, and other nutritious ingredients in her recipes. I've listed many of her cookbooks at the end of this book in Low-Carb Resources.

Last, but not least, you're only going to see net carb counts for these recipes. (The total recipe net carb count is shown in black on the left, and the per serving net carb count is shown on the right.) You're free from counting calories, fat, and cholesterol!

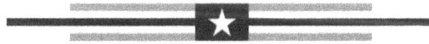

---

24 *Knock Your Socks Off Strawberry Shortcake*
4 Servings   Net Carbs per serving = 6 grams

Ingredients:

1 pound fresh strawberries cleaned and sliced (24)
¼ cup Joseph's clear maltitol sweetener (0)
¼ teaspoon LorAnn Strawberry Naturals flavoring (0)
Land-O-Lakes Sugar-Free Whipped Heavy Cream (0)

Instructions:

Clean and cut up strawberries. Pour Joseph's syrup sweetener in small bowl and stir in LorAnn Strawberry Naturals flavoring. Pour syrup over strawberries and let juices mingle for a few minutes. Stir several times. Serve on top of a Decadent Cake Muffin. Don't spare the whipped heavy cream – you're *not* on a diet. One taste of this oral delight and you'll think you just died and went to heaven! Now, let's get to the cake portion of this dietary decadence.

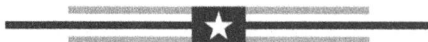

★

18   *Decadent Cake Muffin Recipe*
12 Servings   Net Carbs Per Serving = 1.5 grams

Ingredients:

1 ¼ cups Carbquik (8)

¼ cup ground flax seed (2)

1 ¼ teaspoons baking powder (0)

¼ teaspoon baking soda (0)

½ cup salted butter (1 stick) softened (0)

½ cup *powdered* erythritol (0)

24 drops EZ-Sweetz liquid sucralose - equal to 1 cup sweetener (0)

3 eggs (2)

1 cup grated yellow crookneck squash (2)

2 teaspoons vanilla extract (0)

½ cup regular sour cream (4)

Instructions:

1. Preheat oven to 350 degrees. Spray 12 oversized muffin cups with non-stick oil and set aside.

2. In small bowl, mix together the Carbquik, baking powder, and baking soda, and set aside.

3. In a large bowl, cream the butter until light with an electric mixer on high speed. Add the powdered erythritol and continue beating until the mixture is very light and fluffy. Change the mixer speed to medium. Add the eggs, one at a time, beating well after each addition, then add the vanilla and liquid sucralose. Add squash and stir.

4. Change the mixer speed to low. Alternately beat in the mixed dry ingredients and the sour cream, beginning and ending with the dry ingredients and beating only until combined.

5. Spoon the batter into the prepared muffin cups.

6. Bake for 20-25 minutes. Let the cakes cool on a wire rack for 10 minutes. Gently loosen from the sides, then carefully invert onto the rack and shake to dislodge the cakes. Cool completely before serving or storing.

Variations

V *Almond Cake Muffins*

Instead of 2 teaspoons of vanilla extract, substitute 1 teaspoon vanilla and ½ teaspoon of almond extract.

V *Poppy Seed Almond Cake Muffins* (my personal favorite)

Add 2 teaspoons of poppy seeds to almond cake muffins

V *Cinnamon Swirl Cake Muffins* (or maybe this is my personal favorite, I just can't decide)

To make cinnamon swirl, mix together ¼ cup powdered erythritol, ¼ cup Steel's Nature Sweet (maltitol) Brown Crystals, and 2 teaspoons ground cinnamon. Pour ½ of the batter in each of the 12 muffin cups. Add ½ of the cinnamon swirl mix. Then add the remaining ½ of the batter. Top with remaining ½ of the cinnamon swirl mix. Then spoon 2 tablespoons of melted butter on top of the cinnamon mixture.

Now, we're going to go even further and use this same decadent cake muffin recipe to make some knock your socks off 8 inch square cakes with frosting. Let's start with the frosting.

4 *Decadent Butter Cream Cheese Frosting*
9 Servings   Net Carbs Per Serving = .5 grams

Ingredients:
½ stick of salted butter softened - 1/4 cup (0)

½ block of regular cream cheese softened - 4 ounces (4)

1/3 cup of *powdered* erythritol (granular erythritol will taste gritty) (0)

24 drops of EZ-Sweetz liquid sucralose - equal to 1 cup sweetener (0)

1 teaspoon vanilla extract (0)

Instructions:
Cream butter and cream cheese until well mixed. Add powdered erythritol and stir well. Add liquid sucralose and vanilla extract. Stir until well mixed and smooth.

Variations

V *Chocolate Butter Cream Cheese Frosting*

Melt 2 squares (1 oz each) of unsweetened baking chocolate on defrost in microwave. (Add 8g carbs to total recipe.)

V *Orange Butter Cream Cheese Frosting*

Instead of vanilla extract, substitute 2 teaspoons of LorAnn Orange Natural Flavor Bakery Emulsion.

V *Lemon Butter Cream Cheese Frosting*

Instead of vanilla extract, substitute 2 teaspoons of LorAnn Lemon Natural Flavor Bakery Emulsion.

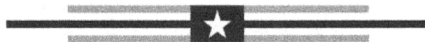

To keep you from flipping back and forth between pages quite so much, I'm going to list the decadent muffin cake muffin recipe again and just modify the baking instructions slightly for the 8 inch square pan.

18 *Decadent 8 Inch Square Cake Recipe*
9 Servings   Net Carbs Per Serving = 2 grams

Ingredients:
1 ¼ cups Carbquik (8)
¼ cup ground flax seed (2)
1 ¼ teaspoons baking powder (0)
¼ teaspoon baking soda (0)
½ cup salted butter (1 stick) softened (0)
½ cup *powdered* erythritol (0)
24 drops EZ-Sweetz liquid sucralose - equal to 1 cup sweetener (0)
3 eggs (2)
1 cup grated yellow crookneck squash (2)
2 teaspoons vanilla extract (0)
½ cup regular sour cream (4)

Instructions:

1. Preheat oven to 350 degrees. Spray 8 inch square pan with non-stick oil and set aside.

2. In small bowl, mix together the Carbquik, baking powder, and baking soda, and set aside.

3. In a large bowl, cream the butter until light with an electric mixer on high speed. Add the powdered erythritol and continue beating until the mixture is very light and fluffy. Change the mixer speed to medium. Add the eggs, one at a time, beating well after each addition, then add the vanilla and liquid sucralose. Add squash and stir.

4. Change the mixer speed to low. Alternately beat in the mixed dry ingredients and the sour cream, beginning and ending with the dry ingredients and beating only until combined.

5. Spoon the batter into the prepared 8 inch square pan.

6. Bake for 30-35 minutes. Cool completely before frosting with basic butter cream cheese frosting.

Variations

V *Banana Nut Cake*

Instead of vanilla extract, substitute 2 teaspoons of LorAnn Banana Naturals flavoring. Add ½ cup of chopped walnuts. When completely cool, frost with Butter Cream Cheese Frosting. (Add 8g carbs to total recipe.)

V *Zucchini Nut Cake*

Substitute zucchini squash for crookneck squash. Add 1 teaspoon cinnamon, ½ teaspoon nutmeg, and ½ cup chopped walnuts. When completely cool, frost with Butter Cream Cheese Frosting. (Add 9g carbs to total recipe.)

V *Pumpkin Pie Spice Cake*

Substitute ½ can (7.5 oz) of Libby's 100% Pure Pumpkin. Add 1 teaspoon ground cinnamon, ½ teaspoon ground ginger, ¼ teaspoon nutmeg, and ¼ teaspoon cloves (optional). Can substitute 2 teaspoons pumpkin pie spice for other spices. When completely cool, frost with Butter Cream Cheese Frosting. (Add 7g carbs to total recipe)

V *Chocolate Cake*

Substitute ½ can (7.5 oz) of Libby's 100% Pure Pumpkin. Melt 2 squares (1 oz each) of unsweetened baking chocolate on defrost in microwave. When completely cool, frost with Chocolate Butter Cream Cheese Frosting. (Add 15g carbs to total recipe.)

V *Orange Cake*

Instead of 2 teaspoons of vanilla extract, substitute 1 tablespoon of LorAnn Orange Natural Flavor Bakery Emulsion and add 1 tablespoon grated orange peel (or 1 teaspoon dried orange peel). When completely cool, frost with Orange Butter Cream Cheese Frosting. Tip: Spice Islands makes dried orange peel.

V *Lemon Cake*

Instead of 2 teaspoons of vanilla extract, substitute 1 tablespoon of LorAnn Lemon Natural Flavor Bakery Emulsion and add 1 tablespoon grated lemon peel (or 1 teaspoon dried lemon peel). When completely cool, frost with Lemon Butter Cream Cheese Frosting. Tip: Spice Islands makes dried lemon peel.

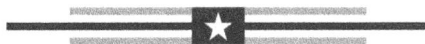

———★———

Now, here's another recipe that gets rave reviews from folks who think they don't like low PSS sweeteners. This is the low PSS coffee cake I was talking about in Chapter 2. After I have my two butter fried eggs and two (Banquet Brown 'N Serve) sausage links, I have a piece of this Raspberry Cream Cheese Coffee Cake. The carb count for this wonderful breakfast? Approximately 9 grams!

Since this recipe calls for preserves and not fresh fruit, you can make this coffee cake any time of the year. There are all sorts of wonderful fruit flavors to choose from, so take your pick. Yes, the fruit preserves do add a lot of carbs, but all fruits are carb intensive.

(The LorAnn Super Strength flavorings are twice as strong as the LorAnn Naturals flavorings. That's why some variations show ½ teaspoon and some show 1 teaspoon. It's not absolutely necessary to use the LorAnn oils, but they add a wonderful fruit sparkle with no additional carbs.)

81 *Raspberry Cream Cheese Coffee Cake*
12 Servings   Net Carbs Per Serving = 7 grams

Ingredients:
2 cups Carbquik (12)
¼ cup ground flax seed (2)
1 cup powdered erythritol (0)
24 drops EZ-Sweetz liquid sucralose - equal to 1 cup sweetener (0)
¾ cup cold salted butter (0)
½ teaspoon baking powder (0)
½ teaspoon baking soda (0)
1 cup regular sour cream (8)
1 egg, beaten (2)
1 teaspoon vanilla extract (0)

½ teaspoon almond extract (0)

1 teaspoon LorAnn Raspberry Super Strength flavoring (0)

FILLING:

1 8 ounce package cream cheese softened (8)

30 drops EZ-Sweetz liquid sucralose - equal to 1¼ cups sweetener (0)

1 egg (2)

1 teaspoon vanilla (0)

1 13.5 ounce jar of Polaner Sugar Free with Fiber Raspberry Preserves (44)

> (Can also use a 10 ounce jar of Nature's Hollow Sugar Free Raspberry Preserves with 28g carbs)

½ cup slivered almonds (4)

Instructions:

1. In a large mixing bowl, combine flour and powdered erythritol. Cut in butter until mixture is crumbly. Remove 1 cup and set aside. To the remaining crumbs, add baking powder and baking soda. Add the sour cream, egg, liquid sucralose, vanilla extract, almond extract, and LorAnn raspberry flavoring; mix well. Spread in a greased 9 inch springform pan.

2. For the filling, in a small bowl, beat cream cheese, liquid sucralose, and egg until blended. Pour over batter; spoon raspberry preserves on top. Sprinkle with almonds and reserved crumbs.

3. Bake at 350 degrees for 45-50 minutes. Let stand for 15 minutes. Carefully run a knife around the edge of pan to loosen; remove sides from pan. Let cool completely or overnight in refrigerator before cutting. (Springform pans have a habit of leaking so put a cookie sheet on the bottom oven rack.)

Variations

V *Strawberry Cream Cheese Coffee Cake*

Substitute 2 teaspoons LorAnn Strawberry Naturals flavoring and a 13.5 ounce jar of Polaner Sugar Free with Fiber Strawberry Preserves or a 10 ounce jar of Nature's Hollow Sugar Free Strawberry Preserves.

V *Apricot Cream Cheese Coffee Cake*

Substitute 1 teaspoon LorAnn Apricot Super Strength flavoring and a 13.5 ounce jar of Polaner Sugar Free with Fiber Apricot Preserves or a 10 ounce jar of Nature's Hollow Sugar Free Apricot Preserves.

V *Blackberry Cream Cheese Coffee Cake*

Substitute 1 teaspoon LorAnn Blackberry Super Strength flavoring and a 13.5 ounce jar of Polaner Sugar Free with Fiber Blackberry Preserves. (Nature's Hollow doesn't offer blackberry preserves.)[10]

V *Peach Cream Cheese Coffee Cake*

Substitute 1 teaspoon LorAnn Peach Super Strength flavoring and a 10 ounce jar of Nature's Hollow Peach Preserves. (Polaner has discontinued its Peach Preserves.)[11]

V *Blueberry Cream Cheese Coffee Cake*

Substitute 2 teaspoons LorAnn Blueberry Naturals flavoring and a 10 ounce jar of Nature's Hollow Blueberry Preserves. (Polaner has discontinued its Blueberry Preserves.)[12]

V *Mountain Berry Cream Cheese Coffee Cake (raspberries, strawberries, blackberries, and blueberries)*

Substitute 1 teaspoon of your choice of LorAnn Super Strength flavoring or 2 teaspoons of LorAnn Naturals flavoring and a 10 ounce jar of Nature's Hollow Mountain Berry Preserves. (Polaner doesn't currently offer this flavor.)[13]

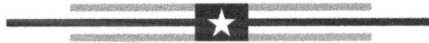

Peggy Tip: *Put powdered erythritol into a shaker bottle and use like regular powdered sugar. It makes your Cream Cheese Coffee Cakes and French toast look absolutely fabulous. Speaking of French Toast...*

21 *Sweet Insanity French Toast*
4 Servings   Net Carbs Per Serving = 5 grams

Ingredients:
2 eggs (2)
½ teaspoon vanilla (0)
½ teaspoon LorAnn Orange Natural Flavor Bakery Emulsion - necessary to experience true insanity (0)
1/3 cup Hood Calorie Countdown 2% milk (1)
4 slices of Sara Lee 45 Calories & Delightful 100% Whole Wheat With Honey bread (18)
2 tablespoons butter (0)
Powdered erythritol (0)
Joseph's All Natural Maple Flavor Sugarfree Syrup (0)
Butter (0)

Instructions:
In small bowl, beat eggs. Add LorAnn orange emulsion (secret ingredient) and milk. Mix well. Pour into a flat bottomed bowl that will accommodate the bread. Dip the bread slices into egg mixture, turning over each slice 3 times. Melt 2 tablespoons butter and cook bread slices until golden brown, about 7 or 8 minutes. Remove from heat; sprinkle with powdered erythritol and cut each piece diagonally. Because the bread is relatively high in PSS, I usually have only one piece of French toast with two fried eggs and bacon. But I drown it in syrup.

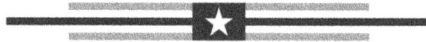

11   *TDF Pancakes*
4 Servings   (8 4"-5" pancakes)   *Net Carbs Per Serving = 3 grams*

Ingredients:
¾ cup Carbquik (4)
¼ cup ground flax seed (2)
1 egg (1)
¾ cup Hood Calorie Countdown 2% milk (3)
2 tablespoons of oil (0)
¼ teaspoon of LorAnn Banana Naturals flavoring -TDF secret ingredient (0)
1 teaspoon cinnamon (0)
1/8 cup finely chopped walnuts (2)
2 tablespoons of oil for cooking (0)
Joseph's All Natural Maple Flavor Sugarfree Syrup (0)
Butter (0)

Instructions:
Mix together dry ingredients. Wisk egg, milk, oil, LorAnn Banana Naturals flavoring, and cinnamon until thoroughly mixed and bubbles. Then add dry ingredients and fold in until only a few lumps remain. Cook until golden brown, about 4-5 minutes. Sometimes I just can't resist adding whipped cream. Yum!

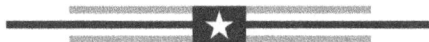

---

18   *Unbelievable low PSS Cookies*
12 Big Cookies   *Net Carbs Per serving = 1.5 grams*

Ingredients:
½ cup salted butter – softened (0)
¾ cup powdered erythritol (0)
1 beaten egg (1)
24 drops EZ-Sweetz liquid sucralose – equal to 1 cup sweetener (0)

2 teaspoons vanilla (0)

1 teaspoon LorAnn Canadian Maple Super Strength flavoring – gives cookies
brown sugar flavor (0)

½ cup grated yellow crookneck squash (1)

1 cup Carbquik (6)

¼ cup ground flax seed (2)

¼ teaspoon soda (0)

½ cup walnuts (8)

Directions:

1. Cream softened butter and powdered erythritol.

2. Beat egg well, and add liquid sucralose, vanilla, and LorAnn flavoring.

3. Add egg mixture to butter mixture and stir well. Add squash.

4. Add sifted dry ingredients, then nuts.

5. Mix all ingredients just until moistened.

6. Drop from tablespoon onto greased cookie sheet and squish down to about ¼ inch thick.

7. Bake at 350 degrees for 12-15 minutes. Inhale deeply as cookies bake.

Variations

V *LorAnn Varieties*

With this basic low PSS cookie recipe, you can invent all sorts of wonderful variations. Take a look at the LorAnn flavorings and you'll see what I mean.

V *Chocolate Chip Nut Cookies*

Add ½ package (4 oz.) Sensato Sugar Free Chocolate Chips (15). (Add 15g carbs to total recipe.)

V *Chocolate-Chocolate Nut Cookies*

Substitute ½ cup of Libby's 100% Pure Pumpkin (3). Melt 1 square (1 oz.) of un-sweetened baking chocolate (2) on defrost in microwave and add to pumpkin mixture. Add ¼ cup unsweetened cocoa powder (8) to flour mixture. (Add 13g carbs to total recipe.)

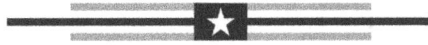

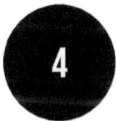

---

4 *Ice Cream Goodies*
½ Cup Serving   *Net Carbs Per Serving = 4 grams*

Safeway Select Watch'n Carbs is a low PSS ice cream. This full-fat rich ice cream is sweetened with Splenda and it tastes wonderful to me. According to my taste testers back in Chapter 4, it tastes better than some of the "leaded" ice creams. At this time, the Colorado Safeway stores only offer two flavors; Vanilla Bean (3g carbs) and Butter Pecan (4g carbs). It comes in 1.5 quart rounds.

But, this li'l old fat lady isn't content with just two ice cream flavors. So, let's look at some ice cream additions that will give us more flavor varieties. In addition to LorAnn flavorings, here are some other really good flavor options for the vanilla ice cream. Just chop up or smash:

- 1 Unbelievable Low PSS Cookie (1.5-2.5)
- 1 Atkins Chocolate Crème Sandwich Cookie (2)
- 1 Reese's sugar-free peanut butter cup candy (.5)
- 1 York sugar-free peppermint patty candy (.5)
- 1 Russell Stover's sugar-free toffee square candy (0)
- 1 Russell Stover's sugar-free peanut butter crunch candy (1)
- 1 Russell Stover's sugar-free peanut brittle candy (1)

You can also make a delicious root beer float and various flavor milkshakes. Just add the vanilla ice cream to A & W Diet Root Beer and to Hood's Calorie Countdown Milk Beverages along with various LorAnn flavorings. One of these days, we may be able to pick from dozens of delectable low PSS ice cream flavors at the grocery store but, today, creativity is the only option. Moving on to smoothies…

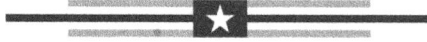

———★———

Since smoothies are all the rage right now, we obviously need a LCHF (Low Carbohydrate High Fat) version for us low PSS folks. I'm also a proponent of the 9 essential amino acids in proteins. So, I plucked out a smoothie called a Power Up! Protein Shake from *The Six-Week Cure for the Middle-Aged Middle* by Michael R. Eades, MD and Mary Dan Eades, MD and doctored it up a bit.[11] Here is my version.

Low PSS Smoothies
6
1 Serving   *Net Carbs Per Serving = 6 grams*

Ingredients:
¾ cup cold water (0)
3 drops EZ-Sweetz liquid sucralose or other sweetener (0)
1 raw egg*(2)
1-2 tablespoons heavy cream (1)
¼ - ½ teaspoon of LorAnn flavoring, see flavor chart a few pages back (0)
1 to 3 scoops of 18g-22g protein low-carb whey protein**(3)
2500 mg leucine - in branch-chain amino acid supplement capsules or powder (0)
2500 mg D-ribose powder – optional (0)
Approximately 1 cup of ice cubes (0)

Instructions:
Place all the ingredients in a blender in the order above and blend on high speed until smooth. Adjust the amount of ice to achieve preferred consistency. Drink immediately. *The Six-Week Cure for the Middle-Aged Middle* has all sorts of good nutritional and medical advice along with some great recipes, so I suggest you might want to invest in the book.

*Drs. Eades suggest a raw egg. If that sounds a little raw, they say that you can buy pasteurized eggs or you can "roll your own" simply by giving a raw egg a 30-60 second dunk (whole in the shell) in boiling water.

** According to Drs. Eades, people under 130 pounds should use one scoop, those 131-180 should use two scoops and those 181 and over should use three scoops. I buy Costco's CytoSport 100% Whey protein in big 6 pound bags. Each scoop has 27 grams of protein and comes in vanilla and chocolate flavors. I use one scoop.

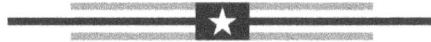

This low PSS pie shell is adapted from Chef Gregory Pryor at Carbquik (Tova Industries) and can be used for everything from sweet desserts to rich egg quiches. It's incredibly simple to make.

15 *Carbquik Pie Shell Recipe*
16 Servings (2 pie crusts)   Net Carbs Per Serving = 1 gram

Ingredients:
2 ½ cups Carbquik (15)
6 ounces by weight of fat of choice, lard shortening or softened butter - I use ¾ cup salted butter (0)
Ice cold water as needed, approximately ¼ cup (0)
Pinch salt - I don't use salt (0)

Instructions:

1. Cut the butter or other fat into the Carbquik with a pastry cutter until a coarse crumb is reached.

2. Mix together the ice water and salt, and sprinkle it over the Carbquik mixture gradually. Combine until a mass forms. Gently gather the dough into a smooth ball.

3.   Divide the dough into two pieces and flatten into disks. Wrap the dough in plastic wrap, and refrigerate for at least 2-24 hours. This process conditions the dough by allowing the Carbquik time to absorb moisture and for the gluten to relax.

4.   When ready to use, bring dough to room temperature and press into a greased 9" pie pan.

5.   To prebake, prick crust all over with a fork and bake at 400 degrees for 15 minutes.

6.   Pie dough will keep for 2-3 days in the refrigerator or 1 month in the freezer.

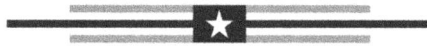

Ok, I think I've just about beaten sweets to a sweet death, so let's move on to some not so sweet menu items. Remember, my goal is to show the "fast food fans" how they can have their cake and eat it too.

Are you a hamburger, hot dog, or bratwurst type? Just substitute Sara Lee's 80 Calories and Delightful buns. They've only got 8-9 net carbs which is less than half of the regular "leaded" buns. Then inspect the hot dog and bratwurst packages with a magnifying glass. Those food processors really like to slip in a little "sugar in sheep's clothing." If your hot dog or bratwurst has added carbs, keep looking.

Now I feel really bad to pop your bubble but, if you're one of the 68.5% of adult Americans who are overweight or obese, you really do need to think about every single carb you consume. Don't cheat. At least not until your scales and blood work tell you that you're in the clear. Remember that Dr. Eric Westman's Duke University Lifestyle Medicine Clinic "No Sugar, No Starch" diet limits you to about 20 carbs per day. Do you really want to blow almost half of your day's allotment on one bun? The answer may be yes, but you want to consciously spend your "carb budget." You need to change your thinking so that your "splurge" is not calories but carbs. By changing your thinking you can help win your health and freedom.

Continuing with the "fast food fans," since your chip and French fry options are pretty limited right now, I've got some other fast food sides that might appeal to you. Maybe coleslaw sounds good? Coleslaw is a piece of cake – figuratively speaking. You've got the regular cabbage varieties and there's even a broccoli slaw in ready to eat 12 ounce bags.

Most of them have approximately two grams of carbs per one cup of slaw so all you need to do is watch out for the sauce. The "unleaded" sauce has only a few ingredients and tastes the same as the "leaded" stuff. Here's a sauce recipe that is inspired by one of Dana's cookbooks.[12] If you want to work just a tiny bit harder, Dana's cookbooks have many more slaw recipes.

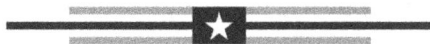

★

---

10   *Low PSS Coleslaw*
4 Servings   *Net Carbs Per Serving = 2.5 grams*

Ingredients:
¼ cup regular mayonnaise (0)
¼ cup regular sour cream (2)
2 teaspoons apple cider vinegar (0)
½ teaspoon prepared mustard (0)
½ teaspoon salt or other low PSS spice mixture (0)
1 drop of EZ-Sweetz liquid sucralose or 2 teaspoons sweetener (0)
12-16 ounce packaged coleslaw (8)

Instructions:
Combine all the ingredients well and then toss with packaged slaw.

Peggy Tip: *You might also want to check out the Smoked Paprika Vinaigrette and Poppy Seed salad dressing recipes below. When you mix them with some mayonnaise and sour cream, they make really good coleslaw sauces, too.*

Now, let me tell you why I'm including salad dressings in this book. First, you should be eating more salads. And second, it's almost impossible to find a prepared salad dressing that doesn't have added "sugar in sheep's clothing." Even non-sweet salad dressings like Ranch and Blue Cheese have the "lead."

Here I'm going to focus on the sweeter salad dressings so that you can see how easy it is to make your "leaded" salad dressings "unleaded." You'll be amazed at the difference a couple of simple ingredient substitutions will make. Here are the ingredient rules.

Substitute EZ-Sweetz liquid sucralose or other sweetener for sugar and low PSS honey for high PSS honey. That's it. Isn't that simple?

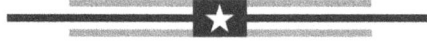

★

---

6 *Low PSS Smoked Paprika Vinaigrette*
12 Servings Net Carbs Per Serving = .5 grams

Ingredients:
½ cup red wine vinegar (0)

1/3 cup low PSS honey (0)

1 tablespoon stone-ground mustard (1)

1 tablespoon lime juice (1)

¾ teaspoon ground black pepper (0)

¾ teaspoon salt (0)

1 ¼ teaspoons smoked paprika (0)

2 cloves garlic (2)

2 tablespoons chopped onion (2)

¼ teaspoon oregano (0)

1 drop of EZ-Sweetz liquid sucralose or 2 teaspoons sweetener – optional (0)

1 cup olive oil (0)

Directions:
Blend the red wine vinegar, low PSS honey, mustard, lime juice, pepper, salt, paprika, garlic, onion, and oregano together in a blender until thoroughly mixed. Drizzle the olive oil into the mixture while blending. Taste. If too tart, add optional sweetener. Chill at least 1 hour before serving.

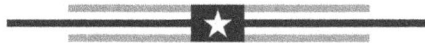

★

Let's do one more low PSS salad dressing.

⑤ *Low PSS Poppy Seed Salad Dressing*
12 Servings Net Carbs Per Serving = .5 grams

Ingredients:

18 drops of EZ-Sweetz liquid sucralose or ¾ cup sweetener (0)

1/3 cup cider vinegar (0)

¼ cup grated onion (4)

1 tablespoon stone-ground mustard (1)

1 teaspoon poppy seeds (0)

½ teaspoon salt (0)

1 cup olive oil (0)

Directions:

In a small bowl, combine the first six ingredients. Slowly add oil, while whisking briskly. Cover and refrigerate until serving. This dressing can also be drizzled over sliced tomatoes and cucumbers and even used as a coleslaw dressing.

Peggy Tip: *These last two salad dressing recipes were inspired by www.allrecipes.com. You should take a look at this web site for more great recipe ideas.*

㉗ *Low PSS Pizza Dough*
4 Servings   Net Carbs Per Serving = 6.5 grams

This is the best low PSS pizza dough recipe I've found. It's one that is posted by Wendy Finn on InfoBarrel. As she says, "…this recipe for low carb pizza dough isn't going to taste like you just picked it up from the Hut, but it tastes really good and will kick those cravings firmly to the curb." You should look at Wendy's post because she's got some really great pictures to go with the instructions. Here's the URL. http://www.infobarrel.com/Low_Carb_Pizza_Crust.

Ingredients:

1 cup of Carbalose flour (19)
1 cup ground flax seed (8)
1½ teaspoons Xanthan Gum - supermarkets usually have this (0)
1 teaspoon salt (0)
2 tablespoons light olive oil (0)
2 teaspoons of yeast (0)
¾ cup of warm water- this amount may vary slightly (0)

Directions:

1. Put all the ingredients except the salt and yeast into a bowl and mix them together. Put the yeast into the bowl on one side, and the salt into the bowl on the other. Now add approximately 3/4 cup of warm water.

2. Mix into a dough using a mixer or food processor, or work it with a spoon at first, and then use your hands to get the mixture into a dough

3. The dough should be quite wet at this stage.

4. Now knead the dough on an oiled work surface that will stop it from sticking.

TIP: Use oil on your work surface when kneading and rolling the dough.

Shaping and Proving:

1. Leave your dough in the bowl, covered with a damp cloth for 15-30 minutes and check to see if it needs any extra flour or water added.

2. Divide into 2 or 3 equal portions and roll into balls. Cover again, and leave in a warm place to rise for at least an hour.

3. Now, the rolling can get messy so I highly recommend you sandwich your dough balls between sheets of wax paper or baking parchment. You get a better finish and you won't have to worry about the dough sticking to your rolling pin.

4. Make sure to roll each ball out thinly, bearing in mind the dough will rise a little in the oven.

Ready for the Toppings:

1. Now that we've made such a wonderful low carb pizza crust, be sure to only use low carb ingredients for the toppings! A regular tomato sauce or passata shouldn't have too many carbs, but be sure to check the ingredients and use sparingly, and of course you can lay on as much cheese and as many herbs as you want! All you have to do now is choose your meat and vegetables wisely.

2. Make sure to heat up a baking sheet in your oven while you are topping up your pizza. Set the oven on as high a temperature as it will go. You should then cook your pizza for around 10 minutes until the crust turns a lovely golden brown.

3. The next part? Just enjoy!

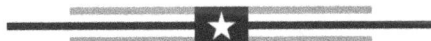

While this li'l old fat lady doesn't currently have a good French fry or baked potato, mashed potatoes are a piece of cake. For a long time, I resisted this recipe because it sounded so horrible to me, but it actually works. The magical ingredient? Cauliflower! Now, come on back. Please stay with me here. You've just got to trust me on this one. I took a recipe from Michael R. Eades, MD and Mary Dan Eades, MD's book, *The Six-Week Cure for the Middle-Aged Middle* and doctored it up a bit. The result is spectacular!

31 *Comfort Cauliflower Mashed Potatoes*
6 Servings   Net Carbs Per Serving = 5 grams

Ingredients:
1 large head cauliflower (16)
4 cloves garlic, mashed (4)
1 block (8 ounces) cream cheese softened (8)
½ stick (1/4 cup) salted butter, melted (0)
¼ cup heavy cream (3)
½ teaspoon salt (0)
¼ teaspoon pepper (0)
1 cup sharp cheddar cheese (0)

Instructions:

1. Wash the cauliflower and trim away tough outer leaves. Cut up cauliflower in ½ inch slices.

2. Place the cauliflower and garlic in a microwave-safe bowl, cover, and microwave on high for 6 minutes. Stir and microwave on high for another 3 minutes. Allow cauliflower to cool slightly.

3. Place the cooked cauliflower and garlic into the workbowl of a food processor. Add the melted butter, cream cheese, cream, salt, and pepper. Process in pulses to start and then on high until smooth. Add more cream if needed to achieve a smooth puree that holds its shape like mashed potatoes. Add cheddar cheese and puree again.

4. Adjust seasonings if needed, and serve.

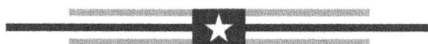

42 *Creamy Cheesy Broccoli Soup*
8 Servings   Net Carbs Per Serving = 5 grams

Ingredients:
    2 large heads of broccoli (4)
    1 recipe of Comfort Cauliflower Mashed Potatoes (31)
    2 cans of Swanson Natural Goodness Chicken Broth (4)
    ¼ (additional) cup heavy cream (3)
    3 (additional) cups sharp cheddar cheese (0)

Instructions:

1. Wash Broccoli and cut in ½ inch slices.

2. Place the broccoli in microwave-safe bowl, cover, and microwave on high for 5 minutes. Stir and microwave on high for another 2 minutes. Allow broccoli to cool slightly.

3. Place the cooked broccoli into the workbowl of a food processor. Process in pulses to start and then on high until broccoli is finely chopped.

4. Make up the recipe of Comfort Cauliflower Mashed Potatoes.

5. Put cooked broccoli and Comfort Cauliflower Mashed Potatoes into a large pot.

6. Add chicken broth and heavy cream. Stir and heat on low.

7. When hot, add cheddar cheese.

8. Adjust seasonings if need, and serve. It's OK if you roll your eyes in delight.

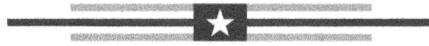

★

Mexican food is also on the menu. Here are two recipes just to prove that you can have your cake and eat it too.

72 *Chicken Fajitas*
8 Servings   Net Carbs Per Serving = 6-9 grams + condiments

Ingredients:
8 boneless skinless chicken thighs or 6 boneless skinless chicken breast halves (0)
½ cup fresh lime juice – most of this juice will not remain with cooked chicken (4)
¾ teaspoon freshly ground black pepper (0)
¾ teaspoon garlic salt (0)
1 large onion, sliced into rings (12)
2 tablespoons butter (0)
1 large green bell pepper, sliced into strips (8)
8 Mission Carb Balance Flour Tortillas (48) or subtract 24 for La Tortilla Factory
    Low Carb High Fiber whole wheat tortillas (24)

Condiments:
Tabasco Green Pepper Sauce or other hot sauce
Guacamole

Pico de gallo or salsa cruda (check carb counts)
Shredded cheddar cheese
Sour cream

Directions:

1. Slice chicken into thin strips.

2. Combine lime juice, black pepper, and garlic salt.

3. In Ziploc bag, marinate chicken in lime juice mixture overnight.

4. In large skillet, sauté onion and green pepper until soft.

5. Grill chicken and then add to vegetable mixture. Stir to mix flavors. Serve with heated tortillas and condiments.

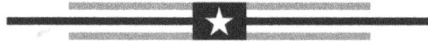

---

30 · *Shrimp Quesadillas*
4 Servings   Net Carbs Per Serving = 7.5 grams + condiments

Ingredients:
½ pound cooked shrimp (6)
2 cups shredded sharp cheddar cheese (0)
4 Mission Carb Balance Flour Tortillas – these taste heavenly when they're fried in butter (24)
4 tablespoons butter (0)

Condiments:
Same as for chicken fajitas

Directions:

1. Cut cooked shrimp into small pieces.

2. Melt 1 tablespoon butter in frying pan and coat both sides of tortilla.

3. Evenly place cut up shrimp on ½ of tortilla then cover shrimp with ½ cup shredded cheese.

4. Fold over tortilla in half and cook on both sides until brown.

5. Serve with condiments.

★

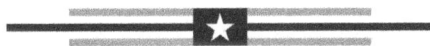

I've saved one of my best recipes for last. Here's a chili recipe that is guaranteed to make your eyes roll. Follow this recipe exactly - no substitutions. You'll make this chili frequently so it's worth buying all the spices.

33

Knock Your Socks Off Chili
8 Servings   Net Carbs Per Serving = 4 grams

Ingredients:

1 ½ pounds ground chuck (0)
1 pound ground pork – the correct stuff will contain only pork and salt (0)
1 cup finely chopped onion (12)
4 cloves chopped garlic (4)
1 12 ounce can low carb light beer (5)
1 8 ounce can Hunt's Tomato Sauce (3)
1 cup water (0)
3 tablespoons chili powder (0)
2 tablespoons ground cumin (0)
1 Knorr beef homestyle stock cup – comes in a package of 4 little cups (4)
2 teaspoons oregano leaves (0)
2 teaspoons paprika (0)

1 drop EZ-Sweetz liquid sucralose or 2 teaspoons sweetener (0)

1 teaspoon cocoa – I use Ghirardelli Natural Unsweetened Cocoa (1)

½ teaspoon dried cilantro (0)

½ teaspoon Louisiana Red Hot Sauce (0)

1 15 ounce can of Eden Organic Black Soy Beans – can find at some health food stores (4)

Directions:

1. Brown beef and pork in large skillet until brown. Remove and set aside in large pot.

2. Add onion and garlic to skillet. Cook and stir until tender. Add to large pot.

3. Add remaining ingredients, mix well, bring to boil, reduce heat, cover, and simmer 2 hours.

4. Serve with warmed Mission Carb Balance Flour Tortilla (6), or La Tortilla Factory Low Carb High Fiber whole wheat tortillas (3) if desired. Did your eyes roll?

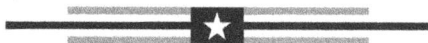

★

PART IV

MARKETING STRATEGIES TO HELP WIN YOUR HEALTH AND FREEDOM

CHAPTER 10

Just One Fourth of a Penny

Do You Believe in Miracles? YES!—Broadcaster Al Michaels

Miracle On Ice – American Hockey's Defining Moment. How the 1980 US Olympic Hockey Team Won Gold.

> The first sign of an upset in the making came at the end of the first period. With time running out, Dave Christian took a long shot. Tretiak stopped it easily, but kicked out a rebound. The Soviet defensemen, expecting the buzzer, seemed to let up on the play. Johnson crashed between them and scored…The Soviets regrouped and were even more dominate in the second period. The Americans managed just two shots on goal, while Craig fended off waves of attackers before Alexander Maltsev scored on a breakaway…In the final 20 minutes, a pillar of the Brooks strategy—speed—came to the fore… Leaving younger, fresher players on the bench, Tikhonov trusted his veterans. Brooks rolled four lines [different players] in quick shifts, taking advantage of tired Soviet legs.[1]

US hockey coach Herb Brooks had changed the game. The Americans were underdogs, but they were competitive.[2] And coach Brooks understood that his team would lose if they played the Soviets' game. Even more profound than Al Michaels' famous call, "Do you Believe in Miracles? *Yes!*" are coach Brooks' brilliant words, "Play your game. Play your game. Play your game. Play your game."[3] Brooks understood that his team needed to change the game to win. They needed to play *their* game, not the Soviets' game.

America is now the fattest nation on earth. And every day, we are losing more of our health and freedom. But we're competitive. We *can* win. However, we need to change the game. We need to turn the kaleidoscope to be able to change our thinking. We need to rise above the ideas of the time. We need to see what *can* be rather than what *is*.

This li'l old fat lady is going to propose a marketing strategy that could change the game to help us Americans regain our health and freedom. Although it focuses on how we can turn the tide of obesity and create new business opportunities, it still involves fundamental change, and some individuals and businesses will feel threatened. Certain individuals will feel uncomfortable about changing their dietary beliefs, and there will be businesses that feel next quarter's earnings might be in jeopardy.

When this happens, you may see behavior that is designed to try and minimize the perceived threat. Two common tactics you'll see are the "cast doubt" routine and the "fundamental-change-hysterical-fear" routine. Here's an example of the "cast doubt" routine. On 60 Minutes, Jim Simon, board member of the Sugar Association states, "The science is not completely clear here." When you see this behavior, just ask yourself what the individual believes or the business thinks it stands to lose if the status quo changes.

Fundamental change is always painful, but this li'l old fat lady's marketing strategy does a lot to minimize the pain. I'm going to itemize the huge benefits that the large majority of Americans can experience. This marketing strategy would:

- Allow Americans to have their cake and eat it, too.

- Turn the tide of obesity in America to help us regain our health and freedom.

- Not force a single American to change his or her beliefs or behavior.

- Minimize the time, effort, cost, and conflict of fundamental change.

- Position America as the world innovator and leader in nutritional enlightenment.

- Help improve the economic vitality of America and even increase our export revenues.

- Address the growing financial burden of the exploding obese, ill baby boomer population.

- Allow America to play America's game.

Now, this li'l old fat lady has just made some pretty big claims, and you may think I'm being a little too optimistic. But the only thing I may be too optimistic about is hoping that

America might just be smart enough to turn the kaleidoscope *before* we've sunk our *Titanic*. Here's my solution in the form of a question. *Is your freedom worth one fourth of a penny?*

The solution is a Freedom Fund. And the cost for the Freedom Fund is only one fourth of a penny.

Now I'm going back to my roots as a marketing professional to describe what I'm talking about. In 1960, the marketer E. Jerome McCarthy proposed a four Ps classification, which has since been used by marketers throughout the world.[4] Here are the four Ps.

- Product—A product is seen as an item that satisfies what a consumer needs or wants.

- Price—The price is the amount a customer pays for the product.

- Promotion—Represents all of the methods of communication that a marketer may use to provide information to different parties about the product.

- Place—Refers to providing the product at a place which is convenient for consumers to access.

Every successful marketing strategy leverages the four Ps to their maximum potential. If any one of the four Ps is changed, it will completely alter the marketing mix[5] and can negatively impact the success of the product. Here's this li'l old fat lady's *Freedom Fund Marketing Strategy*.

MARKETING STRATEGY	DESCRIPTION
Product	A "Freedom Fund" contribution on every PSS or "net carb" that is charged to the final purchaser of each UPC (Universal Product Code) container.
Price	One fourth of a penny per PSS or "net carb."
Promotion	The PSS or "net carb" logo and nutrition information is listed on every UPC container, and a well-designed consumer education program is implemented.
Place	The "Freedom Fund" contribution is applied to all foods and beverages.

The *container* PSS (net carb) logo would be posted on the front of every UPC container in the largest font that is on the label. So, if the largest font on the label is "14," the PSS logo font would also be "14." In addition, the *container* PSS (net carb) number would be posted directly below the "Nutrition Facts" heading on the back of the container. The "Nutrition Facts" label should also include information on the essential amino acids and essential fatty acids. If there's not enough space, how about eliminating some of the stuff that hasn't prevented the obesity epidemic in this country? Here are several logo examples. Just like us humans, the shape of the logo changes from slim to fat as the PSS (net carb) count increases.

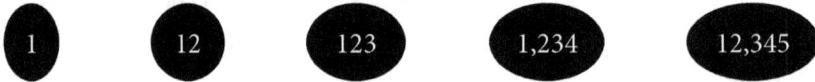

1   12   123   1,234   12,345

Now, let's get into a little more detail. If you'll just hang in here with me, I bet you'll be amazed at how simple this concept is. It's sort of the old Sherlock Holmes saying, "Elementary, my dear Watson."

The Freedom Fund contribution is based on the PSS (net carb) count of the entire *container*, not the "per serving" number. For example, Johnson & Johnson's Splenda sweetener shows a PSS (net carb) count of less than one gram per serving, but there's approximately 24 grams of sugar in sheep's clothing per cup of Splenda. Using simple math (24 times one fourth of a penny), one cup of Splenda will contribute approximately 6¢ to the Freedom Fund. A cup of Cargill's Truvia sweetener with no sugar in sheep's clothing will contribute 0¢ to the Freedom Fund. As a second example, a 12-ounce can of "leaded" Pepsi or Coke with approximately 40 grams of PSS (net carbs) will contribute 10¢ to the Freedom Fund. A 12-ounce can of "unleaded" Diet Pepsi or Diet Coke with zero grams of PSS will contribute 0¢ to the Freedom Fund.

Because the *real* bad boy on the block is causing obesity, diabetes, heart disease, and more, he contributes one fourth of a penny to the Freedom Fund to pay for all the illness and suffering he's causing. Since he's such a bad boy, we just put a tiny price on his head. Then each American and each business gets to decide how much they want to contribute to the Freedom Fund.

As a veteran marketing professional, this li'l old fat lady understands the huge impact that pricing and promotion strategy has on consumer behavior. Here's an example of a pricing and promotion strategy to drive consumer behavior. In a study, *Point-of-Purchase Price and Education Intervention to Reduce Consumption of Sugary Soft Drinks,* conducted at the Brigham and Women's Hospital cafeteria in Boston, Massachusetts, the sales of regular soft drinks declined by 26% during the price increase (of 35%) phase. This reduction in sales persisted throughout the study period, with an additional decline of 18% during the combination of price increase and education campaign phase.[6]

Something as cheap as a one fourth of a penny Freedom Fund contribution along with a prominently displayed PSS (net carb) logo and a well-designed consumer education program can literally turn the tide of obesity in America. Yes, it can! Malcolm Gladwell's book *The Tipping Point*[7] provides many real-world examples of how one well-placed lever can move the world. That's what the Freedom Fund is—a well-placed lever. It's sort of like Sherlock Holmes' magnifying glass that will allow Americans to clearly see the *real* bad boy on the block.

So, what's the daily cost to the average American? Well, it depends. If you're like me, the cost is less than 10¢ a day. The labels on our processed foods recommend 300 grams of carbohydrate for someone consuming 2,000 calories a day and 375 grams for someone consuming 2,500 calories a day. That would mean 75¢–94¢ per day. This li'l old fat lady believes most Americans would be much healthier and leaner if the average person's PSS (carb) intake was less than 100–200 grams. That translates to less than 25¢-50¢. You can't buy much of anything these days that costs less than 50¢.

In comparison, one gallon of gasoline has 46.6¢ hidden in the price in California. And the price of hard liquor in the state of Washington conceals $26.45 in the price. Then there's $2.34 per gallon of wine in North Carolina, and $1.05 per gallon of beer in Alabama. A pack of cigarettes in Rhode Island has $3.46 hidden in the price.[8] While all of these examples are "nontransparent" or hidden, the Freedom Fund contribution needs to be "transparent." Why? Because we want to clearly see the *real* bad boy on the block. We want to put a great big magnifying glass on the *real* culprit.

So, whether the daily Freedom Fund contribution is 10¢, 50¢, or a buck, the cost per person is extremely small. Don't think that Americans can afford it? According to the Associated Press, Americans bought nearly $1.5 billion worth of lotto tickets for a single $640 Mega Millions jackpot.[9] What's driving folks to spend all this money to buy lotto tickets? Hope. That's precisely what this li'l old fat lady is peddling, too. Hope for Americans.

What is the Freedom Fund? It's a fund that comes directly *from* Americans and directly *to* Americans. It's not a fund to bail out special-interest groups like the banking and mortgage industries or the automotive industries. It's not a fund to pay for pork barrel projects. No, it's a fund to pay for the scientifically unsound US government nutritional policy that has been in place since Friday, January 14, 1977, when Senator George Mc-Govern announced the publication of the first *Dietary Goals for the United States*. It's a fund to help offset the $300 billion[10] cost associated with a Medicare SGR (sustainable growth rate) formula repeal so that our medical doctors, hospitals, and pharmaceutical company can be paid appropriately.

At least 95% of the Freedom Fund should go directly back to Americans. No more than 5% of the fund should be used for making sure there are no cheaters. And when the cheaters are identified, they need to end up paying more than 5%. The law should dictate that the funds can never be used for any other program or for any other purpose. So, the Freedom Fund is truly *from* Americans *to* Americans.

Since it can take 35 years for the *real* bad boy on the block to rear his ugly head, the Freedom Fund is for preventing the economic collapse that is likely going to happen due to the exploding obese, sick, baby boomer population. By using the Freedom Fund to pay for Medicare health care coverage and prescription medications, our medical doctors, hospitals, and pharmaceutical companies can be paid appropriately. And all the headlines that talk about Medicare being back on the brink over 27.4% cuts to doctors and increasing Medicare costs should disappear. Headlines like *Medicare back on the brink over cuts to doctors*[11] and *Medicare costs to reduce Social Security increase.*[12]

With an estimated 311,591,917[13] Americans contributing a tiny amount each and every day for the *real* bad boy on the block, we could put a great big Band-Aid on the $464 billion Medicare budget (51% of the $911 billion Health and Human Services 2011 budget).[14] How big would this Band-Aid be? Well, the size of the Band-Aid depends upon how much we're consuming of the *real* bad boy on the block. So, let's take a look.

The labels on our processed foods recommend 300 grams of carbohydrate for someone consuming 2,000 calories a day and 375 grams for someone consuming 2,500 calories a day. That would mean 75¢–94¢ per day. But, based on the 2004 *American Journal of Clinical Nutrition* study titled "An increased consumption of refined carbohydrates and the epidemic of type 2 diabetes in the United States: an ecologic assessment,"[15] this li'l old fat lady believes that carbohydrate consumption may actually exceed 500 grams a day. In 1995 it was about 500 grams a day, so, based on the ever increasing overweight and obesity rates in America, it's probably even higher in 2012. To refresh your memory, here's the chart I showed you back in chapter 3, "The *Real* Bad Boy on the Block."

OBESITY IN AMERICA

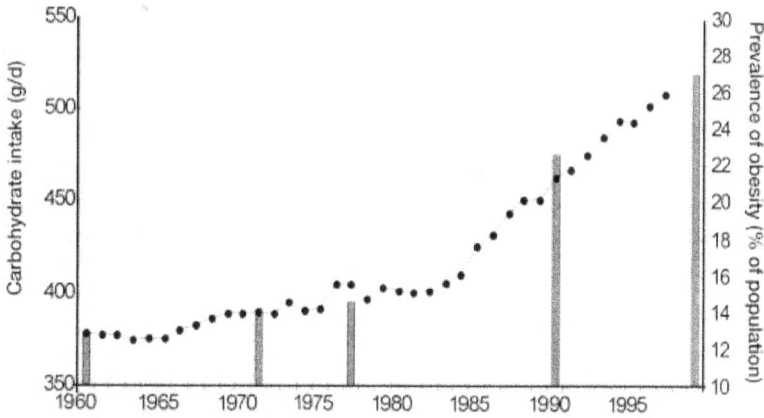

Figure 5. Increasing prevalence of obesity [BMI (in kg/m2) > 30; vertical bars] in the United States between 1960 and 1997 with increasing carbohydrate intake.[16]

So, for argument's sake, let's use 500 grams of carbohydrate intake a day to see how big the Band-Aid would be: 500 X ¼ cents = $1.25. Next you multiply that by 311,591,917 = $389,489,896 X 365 = $142,163,812,040. Shortened up, that means an annual Freedom Fund contribution of $142 billion, which is more than 30% of the 2011 $464 billion Medicare budget. Just one fourth of a penny for the *real* bad boy on the block and Bam! The baby boomer Medicare problem isn't booming so loudly any more.

Still not enough going into the Freedom Fund? Well, here's another potential Freedom Fund source. It's America's dogs and cats, who have apparently become lazy gluttons, too. Here's what the American Society for the Prevention of Cruelty to Animals (ASPCA) has to say: "Obesity is an extremely common problem in pets, and, as with humans, can be detrimental to the health of a dog [or cat]. The overweight pet has many added stresses upon his body and is at an increased risk of diabetes, liver problems, and joint pain."[17]

According to www.petmd.com, "A recent survey indicates over 50% of America's pet population is overweight or obese." PetMD even categorizes our obese dogs into four groups, "Nibbler, Beggar, Good Dog, and Gourmet Dog."[18] The Humane Society approximates that Americans own 78.2 million dogs and 86.4 million cats, or 164.6 million dogs and cats.[19] Over 50% would mean that more than 82.3 million precious American family pets are overweight or obese.

Just like us humans, our pets are supposedly consuming too many calories and not exercising enough. The ASPCA even talks about "Owner Behavior Modification."[20] But guess what America's pets are eating? The same PSS (carbohydrate) rich diet we humans are eating! While pet food doesn't state the PSS counts, the biggest (first) ingredient in most dry pet foods is PSS in some form of corn. So, this li'l old fat lady is willing to bet that many of our beloved pets are also victims of the *real* bad boy on the block.

Why do most of our pet food manufacturers put so much of the *real* bad boy on the block in our beloved pet's food? Because it's cheap! By invoking a tiny one fourth of a penny Freedom Fund contribution per gram of PSS (net carbohydrates) in our pet foods, pet owners can bet that they would see all sorts of *New & Improved!* pet foods. This li'l old fat lady also bets Americans would see their 82.3 million beloved overweight or obese dogs and cats start to slim down and become more healthy. How much Freedom Fund contributions would increase is anyone's guess. But, just to put something out there, let's say 25¢ per day per 164.6 million pets. That adds up to an annual Freedom Fund contribution of $15 billion. It's not a huge amount, but the lives of our pets would be greatly improved.

Don't believe me? Well, here's a subject matter expert who has all the right suffixes. Mary Vernon, MD, FAAFP, FASBP, CMD, is a recognized bariatric (weight loss) expert who utilizes low carbohydrate dietary strategies to heal a multitude of clinical ailments in her human patients. She also has 40-plus years of experience training animals, including dogs, cats, horses, and one chicken. Dr. Vernon has participated in the training of 10 nationally ranked agility dogs, including the number two beagle (two years) and number one Norfolk Terrier (eight years).[21] When asked what she feeds her dogs her answer is, "My dogs eat the highest protein dog food that's available."[22]

OK, back to us humans. Now this li'l old fat lady realizes what she's really proposing and I'm sure the big boys at the fast food joints and processed foods companies like General Mills, Kellogg's, and Kraft get it, too. When the average American starts to see the *real* bad boy on the block on his or her grocery store receipts and fast food bills, he or she is going to start running from this bad boy. This li'l old fat lady understands that this fundamental change is really scary and upsetting to big business, but there really *is* lots of opportunity to generate more revenue for next quarter's earnings. Just think, *New & Improved!*

Let me give you an example. A McDonald's Big Mac has 45 grams of PSS (carbs).[23] Most of these carbs are from the bun. By using a product like Carbquik, the bun net PSS count could easily be reduced to about three grams. Then, get the "leaded" sweetener out of the special sauce, and bingo! *New &Improved!* The trick is to make the *New & Improved!* "unleaded" Big Mac look and taste as good or better than the old "leaded" Big Mac. We're not talking diet food here. You give up PSS, but you get calories, fat, personal freedom, and health back. Because the *New & Improved!* Big Mac only has about four grams of PSS (net carbs), the customer only contributes a penny to the Freedom Fund. And McDonald's should see more customers opening their wallets because the fast food guilt trip is gone. *Nobody is on a diet anymore!*

Pizza joints like Pizza Hut, Domino's Pizza, Little Caesars Pizza, and others really have it easy. Fix the pizza dough, get the added *real* bad boy out of the sauce, and you're home free. The cheese and most of the other toppings won't generate a dime for the Freedom Fund. The Taco Bells and other Mexican fast food joints have a little more challenge, but I'm certain you can come up with a *New & Improved!* menu, too.

Fried chicken joints like Kentucky Fried Chicken, Church's Chicken, and Popeyes Louisiana Kitchen just need to make their "core product" fried chicken. There's only three grams of PSS (carbs) but 10 grams of essential protein contained in a Church's fried chicken leg.[24] But the fat they fry the chicken in needs to be free of trans fats. They could even cook their *New & Improved!* fried chicken in something like organic lard. Yes, lard. At least that's what low carb weight loss experts Michael R. Eades, MD, and Mary Dan Eades, MD, say in their book, *The Six-Week Cure for the Middle-Aged Middle.*[25] Then, get the *real* bad boy out of the fries, coleslaw, and drinks, and you're good to go. Just think, health conscious Americans lining up outside your doors demanding world class fried chicken!

Now, I know there are many health conscious folks out there who will be completely outraged. Hamburger, pizza, and chicken joints! It's *all* horrible junk food! Yes, right now it's really in vogue to bash the fast food industry. But the only thing horrible about the fast food joints is the obscene quantities of highly processed sugars and starches in their food. Don't believe this li'l old fat lady? Here's a statement from Mary Vernon, MD. Again, she's a recognized bariatric (weight loss) expert who utilizes low carbohydrate dietary strategies to heal a multitude of clinical ailments in her patients. "The worst hamburger we have is better than what happens to people when they have their legs amputated from peripheral arterial disease from diabetes….The worst hamburger we have is better than the highly processed sugars and starches, in my opinion."[26] So, even "pink slime" hamburger meat is better than the "leaded" buns, pizza dough, mashed potatoes, french fries, sodas, and sugary desserts that the fast food joints are currently peddling.

However, it's not just the fast food joints who are loading processed sugars and starches high on our plates. The elite five-star gourmet restaurants are doing exactly the same thing. First, they serve that expensive Mesclun and Tamari Salad with Coccodrillo Ciabatta bread. Next, they follow it up with Olathe Sweet Corn Chowder, Grilled Scallion Country Potato, Farro and Mung Bean Jeera Rice, and Linguini Corsara with Shrimp. Then comes the rich, decadent Bittersweet Chocolate Molten, Hot Sticky Toffee Pudding Cake, and Warmed Banana Bread with Vanilla Ice Cream and Caramel Sauce. Instead of a Big Gulp soda, they serve the Detox-Tini, a concoction of Van Gogh Acai-Blueberry Vodka, lime, pomegranate juice, and a touch of St. Germain Elderflower Liqueur. So, yes, from a highly processed sugars and starches standpoint, the expensive five-star restaurants are no better than the greasiest fast food joints out there.

Now you big fast food guys and other big business eateries shouldn't complain about the Freedom Fund. The federal government already requires that you list the nutritional content of all your foods. Just add up the PSS (net carb) content on your nutrition labels and multiply that number by one fourth of a penny. Add the Freedom Fund contribution to your existing customer receipt and there you go. Your customer has the freedom to eat what he or she wants as long as he or she is willing to contribute one fourth of a penny to the Freedom Fund. Since the *real* bad boy on the block causes obesity, diabetes, heart disease, and other nasty illnesses, the folks who don't want to change should be required to "carry their own weight."

The grocery stores shouldn't complain either, because almost all of the food items in the store already have a UPC (Universal Product Code) on the back. With our current computer technology, all we have to do is input the total *container* PSS (net carb) number into the data base and do something as simple as put that number in parentheses as part of the product description on the receipt. Then, at the bottom of the receipt, the total PSS (net carb) number is added up and multiplied by one fourth of a penny. All of the PSS logos on all of the processed food containers should add up to what's on the bottom of the receipt. If your customer wants to buy obscene amounts of the *real* bad boy on the block, he or she shouldn't mind contributing one fourth of a penny to the Freedom Fund. Again, Americans should be required to "carry their own weight."

Now, let's go back to General Mills, Kellogg's, and Kraft for a moment. I know you big boys and the wheat, corn, rice, and potato farmers are already putting on your battle fatigues, but can we sit down for a moment and talk? There *is* a way for all you folks to win at this game, too, but you need to think outside the box. We really do need to turn the kaleidoscope to see the enormous possibilities.

This li'l old fat lady is looking at numerous headlines and scientific articles that can change the game. Not just for America, but for the world. Unfortunately, some of these headlines are for work that is currently being done in India, so we need to get our backsides in gear. To help establish America as the world innovator and leader in nutritional enlightenment, we need to adopt the Specialized *"Innovate or Die"* motto to quickly move us forward. Here are some example headlines and articles we should all be paying attention to. *Remember, good quality protein with the nine essential amino acids and essential fats helps keep us alive, healthy, and normal weight.*

- *High-protein, low-carb corn developed.* "Daniel Gallie, professor of biochemistry at UC (University of California) Riverside in the United States, has successfully doubled the protein and oil content of corn grain, a discovery that could significantly add value to the crop and benefit corn producers…It could provide a good source of protein for those that depend on grain as their primary source of nutrients…It's basically the same corn, except that it is protein-rich and starch-poor – something that, if applied to sweet corn, would appeal to a large number of weight-conscious people in this country who are interested in low-carb diets and who normally avoid corn in their diets."[27]

- *High-protein rice that fights drowsiness, global warming.* "Conventional rice has barely 7–8 percent protein, while the high-protein rice (HPR) contains as much as 14-15 percent protein. 'This would also mean that the carbohydrate content would be low.' Shailaja Hittalmani, professor at the department of genetics and plant breading at the University of Agricultural Sciences (in India), states that the HPR is not genetically modified but a hybrid. It also uses 60% less water to grow."[28]

- *Get set for potatoes high on protein.* "Scientists at the National Institute for Plant Genome Research in New Delhi (India) are planning to seek regulatory approval for commercial cultivation of a high protein potato that they have developed through genetic modification. Nicknamed 'protato,' the protein packed genetically modified (GM) potato contains 60% more protein than a wild-type potato and has increased levels of several amino acids…The

AmA1 [gene] has great agricultural importance because it is a well-balanced protein in terms of amino acid composition, possessing even better values than recommended by the World Health Organization for a nutritionally rich protein."[29] Yes, this li'l old fat lady realizes that many folks vehemently object to GM foods. But, they're probably here to stay. In 2006, the United States alone grew 53% of the global transgenic crops.[30] But, if you still don't like the idea of GM, how about the next potato example?

- *Low-carb potato hits the market for grateful carb watchers.* "Dr. Chad Hutchinson, from Florida University, and HZPC, a Dutch seed company, have been working on developing a new carb-friendly potato for years. Hutchinson said this new spud is the future of the potato. He also added that this new potato is the result of breeding rather than genetic tinkering… It looks pretty much the same as any ordinary potato; it is yellow and waxy with a smooth skin. Researchers say that its flavor is exceptional."[31] This potato is currently being sold primarily in Florida under the SunLite brand.

- *Export markets paying premiums for high protein wheat.* According to Frayne Olson, a North Dakota State University crops economist, "With protein spreads, the last couple of years have been just wild."[32] What's happening is that a significant amount of the premium-priced high-protein wheat grown in America is being exported to other countries rather than being used to produce our own processed foods. We export the nutritious, high-protein wheat at premium prices and keep the low-priced, high-carbohydrate wheat that causes obesity, diabetes, high blood pressure, diabetes, and more to feed our own American citizens.

So, processed food industry and wheat, corn, rice, and potato growers, rather than put on your battle fatigues, how about rolling up your sleeves and figuring out how to cash in on *New & Improved!*? Remember, eating good quality essential proteins and essential fats while avoiding the *real* bad boy on the block will result in a leaner and healthier customer. And, right now, there's 200-million-plus overweight and obese Americans who will beat a path to your door if you will help them become normal weight and healthy. This li'l old fat lady would think she died and went to heaven if she could order up a *New & Improved!* Big Mac and fries at McDonald's that didn't cause her pancreas to poison her.

But, speaking to the fast food and processed food industries, this is not just about *New & Improved!* Here's the reality. If we don't turn the obesity epidemic tide in this country pretty soon, fewer and fewer people are going to have enough money to buy all your processed "leaded" foods. Here's what a study by the *Journal of Epidemiological and Community Health* has to say in a research article titled *Wider income gaps, wider waist-bands? An ecological study of obesity and income inequality.* "Obesity, diabetes mortality, and calorie consumption were associated with income inequality in developed countries"[33] In other words, the fatter you get, the less money you have to spend. So, what we've got going right now is a lose-lose situation.

So, why don't you processed food industry folks just figure out how you can make more money and, at the same time, help stop the downward economic spiral that we're currently in. Perhaps we Americans should take a lesson from Detroit. During the 1970s and 1980s, while our big American automakers were sitting around with their thumbs up their nose producing inferior automobiles, Japan came in and cleaned up. America is about to repeat this same scenario with our processed food industries. Only this time it may be India that cleans up with its superior strains of high-protein potatoes and rice.

This li'l old fat lady believes that America has the most favorable factor condition on planet Earth: 309,607,601 acres of rich "harvested cropland" (that's a USDA term)[34] to produce the most superior high-protein, low-carbohydrate wheat, corn, rice, and potatoes for Americans and for the rest of the world. If we would just get our backsides in gear, America could begin producing more profitable and more nutritious *New & Improved!* crops for our citizens as well as generate huge export revenue streams. This really could happen. But we must turn the kaleidoscope to be able to raise ourselves above the ideas of the time. We need to see what *can* be rather than what *is*.

Now, even if America implemented this li'l old fat lady's Freedom Fund Marketing Strategy tomorrow, it would still be several decades before some folks changed their beliefs and eating habits. That's just how we humans are. In the technology world, this type of change is called a Discontinuous Innovation, and there's a classic bell-shaped curve associated with the rate of adoption. But it's a special bell that has cracks. Geoffrey A. Moore is the author of a book called *Crossing the Chasm*. Its focus is on "Marketing and Selling High-Tech Products to Mainstream Customers," but the same rules also apply to all fundamental changes. Here are Geoffrey Moore's two bell-shaped curves.[35]

Technology Adoption Life Cycle

The *Revised* Technology Adoption Life Cycle

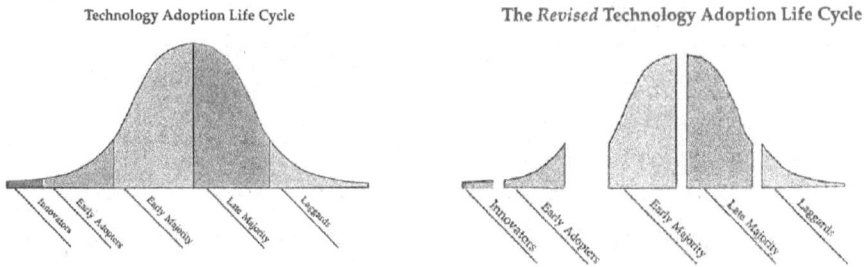

Let me give you an example of Continuous Innovation vs. Discontinuous Innovation. Cooking stoves originally used some sort of fossil fuel like natural or propane gas, wood, or oil. Later, the electric stove was introduced. The electric stove is an example of a Continuous Innovation. In both cases, consumers use a heat source to cook their food so they don't have to radically change their thinking or behavior to use an electric stove. Then came the microwave oven. It's a Discontinuous Innovation because it requires consumers to radically change the way they cook food. There's no physical heat source. The rules of cooking are completely changed. And early on there was all sorts of "fundamental-change-hysterical-fear" about how microwave ovens were going to kill us all. Ditto with Dr. Atkins's ideas almost 40 years ago. Back then it was the "fundamental-change-hysterical-fear" routine towards a diet that eliminated excessive carbohydrates as "nutritionally unsound and potentially dangerous."

Now, there's a reasonably good chance that a Discontinuous Innovation will fall into one of the bell's cracks. Geoffrey Moore's term for the crack is *Chasm*. That is exactly what happened with the low carb craze in 2003, partly because the consumer marketing message was negative. *Eliminate* carbs, we were told. That was *after* we consumers had already been told to eliminate fat, cholesterol, red meat, eggs, cheese, and calories. Of course consumers would have none of it!

But this li'l old fat lady's Freedom Fund Marketing Strategy message is different. My message is, *"If you give up carbs, you get back fat, cholesterol, red meat, eggs, cheese, calories, ice cream, cake, and much more. You also get your personal freedom and health back."* And I show big business how they can make more money and improve next quarter's earnings at the same time. The Freedom Fund is a bridge (or lever or tipping point or magnifying glass) that runs over each chasm to help ensure we will eventually get to the other side of the obesity epidemic to regain America's health and freedom.

Now, if you look back in recent history, the Discontinuous Innovation market adoption rates for the microwave oven, personal computer, cell phones, voice messaging, high-speed Internet, and high-definition TVs invariably began as a trickle but then eventually ballooned into increasingly larger consumer demand. One of my big challenges as a marketing professional was to try and rein in the overly optimistic corporate executives in the large company I worked for. They *always* overestimated early market demand for Discontinuous Innovations.

The beauty of this Freedom Fund Marketing Strategy is that while many Americans are hesitating, we're paying one fourth of a penny. So, the largest contributions to the Freedom Fund are up front, while the sick, obese, baby boomer population is peaking. This li'l old fat lady's school-of-hard-knocks best guess is that it would take at least 20 years to get some Americans to finally accept that excessive carbohydrates are truly the *real* bad boy on the block and thereby significantly lower their carbohydrate consumption.

Why such a pessimistic forecast? Because we're talking about a *real* bad boy on the block who may not raise his head for 35 years. Because we're talking about fundamental change *and* addiction. The closest thing to carbohydrate addiction may be cigarette addiction. So, let's look at cigarette consumption in this country. Some of the CDC cigarette usage records date all the way back to 1964. As a general rule, there has been a slow but constant decline over time. Here's some summary information.

Percent of Adults Who Were Current Smokers[36]

Year	1965	1974	2009	% Change 1965–2009
Total	42.4%	37.1%	20.6%	-51.4%
Male	51.9%	43.1%	23.5%	-54.7%
Female	33.9%	32.1%	17.9%	-47.2%

Now, here's a summary of another CDC table that is even more illuminating. While the number of smoking Americans has dropped by 51.4%, the average number of cigarettes smoked per day among the remaining 51.4% has dropped even more. This CDC data goes back to 1974.

Percent of Adults Who Smoke by the Number of Cigarettes Smoked Daily[37]

Number of Cigarettes Smoked Per Day	1974	2009	% Change 1974–2009
Fewer than 15	31.6%	57.6%	82.3%
15–24	43.2%	32.7%	-24.3%
More than 24	25.3%	9.0%	-64.4%

As you can see, it's taken a long time for many folks to change their smoking habits. Over a 35-year time frame, we've seen a 51.4% decline in the number of smokers and a 64.4% decline in heavy smoking (over 24 cigarettes per day) among the remaining smokers. But if it's taken 35 years to produce these results for smoking, why does this li'l old fat lady believe it may only be 20 years for carbohydrate addiction? Because, with our new "unleaded" sweeteners that are made from corn and other plants and additional low PSS (low carb) food options, we don't really need to give up our carbohydrate addiction. We just need to change our high PSS diet to a low PSS diet.

But this is still a fundamental change, and some folks will resist it more than others. So it may take 20 years for the Late Majority and Laggard Americans to finally accept that the earth is not at the center of the universe and for the processed food industry to finally get its act completely together. Because I believe this point is so important, here's this li'l old fat lady's prediction one more time.

Peggy Prediction: *Based upon my own weight loss journey, I found it very easy to break the physical metabolic addiction to excessive sweets and carbohydrates. But, like alcoholism, nicotine, and other addictions, fixing the disturbances in my brain's reward circuits proved to be very difficult. So, I predict that, after consuming excessive carbohydrates for many decades, the brain's abnormal addicted desire for carbohydrates and the taste of sweet is almost impossible to break. That's why I have my cake and eat it too.*

OK, let's move on. When designing marketing strategies, there's always a hole. The strategy does have a hole, but this li'l old fat lady has thought long and hard about a way to plug the hole so that some of the benefits of the Freedom Fund don't leak out and away from the obese, ill baby boomer and all the other Americans.

Here's the hole. It's quality control on the nutrition label. How do we know if the nutrition label on the back of all our foods is accurate? If the PSS (net carb) count is understated on the label, big business wins by making their high carb product cost less, and the rest of us Americans end up taking it in the shorts. With one fourth of a penny at stake, unless we figure out a way to eliminate any upside for cheating, there are always a few who will cheat by understating the PSS count on the nutrition label. Remember, the Freedom Fund contribution is based on the PSS (net carb) count of the entire UPC container. The lower the PSS count on the UPC container, the lower the Freedom Fund contribution.

In addition to cheating, "in the US, food manufacturers are permitted an error of plus or minus 20% when stating carbohydrate [and other Class II nutrients] content on product nutrition labels."[38] The full FDA language around the "80/120 rule" can be found in FDA Regulation 21CFR101.9(g).[39] So, the Class II (carbohydrate) nutrient variance allowed by the FDA is 40%! This li'l old fat lady believes that this winky-winky FDA policy needs to stop. If Americans can figure out how to get a man on the moon, we can figure out how to accurately calculate the carbohydrate content in our foods.

Now, I'm going to show you an example of what I'm talking about. I chose Victoria Products because they are "good guys" who understand that long-term, excessive carbohydrate consumption will cause obesity, high blood pressure, heart disease, and more. Here's what their website states: "High-carbohydrate diet causes the pancreas to produce large amounts of insulin, and if this happens for many years in a genetically predisposed person, the insulin receptors throughout the body become resistant to insulin. Because insulin's action is to drive glucose into the cells, this results in chronic hyperglycemia, also known [as] 'high blood sugar.' A large portion of this sugar is stored as fat resulting in obesity. Excess insulin also causes hypertension, and helps initiate the sequence of events in the arterial wall which leads to atherosclerosis and heart disease."[40] Victoria is one of my heroes because they "get it" and produce foods that will help keep Americans slim and healthy. They even post the carb content information of many of their products on their website.

Victoria produces a wonderful marinara sauce called White Linen Collection Gourmet Pasta Sauce. Most of the time Costco carries this mouthwatering sauce at a very reasonable price, and I always make sure I have some on hand. For a time, the nutrition label on this sauce showed total carbohydrates at four grams, dietary fiber at two grams, and sugars at three grams per half-cup serving. The current way to get to the PSS (net carb) count is subtract dietary fiber and any sugar alcohols from total carbohydrate. In the case of this marinara sauce, this would result in a PSS count of two grams. But, what about the sugars of three grams? The math just doesn't add up.

Then, a short time later, I purchased another jar of the same marinara sauce. Here's the nutrition label information: total carbohydrate, eight grams; dietary fiber, one gram; sugars, five grams per half cup serving. That would result in a PSS (net carb) count of seven grams. Here are the labels.

Nutrition Facts	
Serving Size 1/2 Cup (113g)	
Servings Per Container 10	
Amount Per Serving	
Calories 70	Calories from Fat 35
	% Daily Value *
Total Fat 4g	6%
Saturated Fat 1g	5%
Trans Fat 0g	
Cholesterol 0mg	0%
Sodium 380mg	16%
Total Carbohydrate 4g	1%
Dietary Fiber 2g	8%
Sugars 3g	
Protein 2g	4%
Vitamin A 30% • Vitamin C 2%	
Calcium 2% • Iron 8%	
*Percent Daily Values are based on a 2,000 calorie diet.	

INGREDIENTS: IMPORTED ITALIAN TOMATOES, PURE ITALIAN OLIVE OIL, FRESH WHITE ONIONS, FRESH CHOPPED BASIL, FRESH GARLIC, SEA SALT AND SPICES.
WHITE LINEN COLLECTION MARINARA SAUCE IS A CHOLESTEROL FREE FOOD
REFRIGERATE AFTER OPENING
SHAKE WELL BEFORE USING

Victoria
Made In a Green Facility
Green with Sustainable Packaging

Victoria
SINCE 1929
A FAMILY OWNED BUSINESS
DISTRIBUTED BY:
VICTORIA PACKING CORP.
BROOKLYN, NY 11236
www.victoriapacking.com
MADE IN U.S.A.

Nutrition Facts	
Serving Size 1/2 Cup (113g)	
Servings Per Container 10	
Amount Per Serving	
Calories 70	Calories from Fat 35
	% Daily Value *
Total Fat 4g	6%
Saturated Fat 1g	5%
Trans Fat 0g	
Cholesterol 0mg	0%
Sodium 380mg	16%
Total Carbohydrate 8g	1%
Dietary Fiber 1g	4%
Sugars 5g	
Protein 2g	4%
Vitamin A 8% • Vitamin C 4%	
Calcium 2% • Iron 8%	
*Percent Daily Values are based on a 2,000 calorie diet.	

INGREDIENTS: IMPORTED ITALIAN TOMATOES, PURE ITALIAN OLIVE OIL, FRESH WHITE ONIONS, FRESH CHOPPED BASIL, FRESH GARLIC, SEA SALT AND SPICES.
WHITE LINEN COLLECTION MARINARA SAUCE IS A CHOLESTEROL FREE FOOD
REFRIGERATE AFTER OPENING
SHAKE WELL BEFORE USING

Victoria
SINCE 1929
A FAMILY OWNED BUSINESS
DISTRIBUTED BY:
VICTORIA FINE FOODS
BROOKLYN, NY 11236
www.victoriafinefoods.com
MADE IN U.S.A.

So, between these two labels for the same marinara sauce, the PSS count varies widely. One label has a "net carb" count of two grams per half-cup serving, and the other label has a "net carb" count of seven grams per half-cup serving. That's a lot of difference. How could this happen? While it could be caused by sloppy nutritional testing, I suspect that it may be caused by the carbohydrate differences in the tomatoes. One production batch will have a different carb count than another. While this example shows extreme carb count differences between two production batches, some variance between production batches will most likely be the norm. Victoria gets a gold star because they aggressively monitor the carb content of their foods.

Here's a way to plug this hole. All processed foods carry "production batch" information in the form of that little indecipherable coding on the container. For example, one of the Victoria jar lids states, "BEST BY 10/11/2014 18:50 KOSHER PARVE VGBEA S." The other jar lid states, "BEST BY 11/08/2014 23:30 KOSHER PARVE VMBBA N." All processed food companies keep records of their production batches so that they can recall their product if some sort of problem is identified. All of the processed foods carry the Universal Product Code (UPC), and all the UPCs are "owned" by a business that makes money by selling the processed food. The UPC codes are issued by the Uniform Code Council (UCC).

Here's this li'l old fat lady's recommendation to stop any cheating. We put all of the UPC codes for every food or beverage product that we Americans consume into an electronic hopper, sort of like those Bingo or Powerball hoppers. Each day a certain number of the UPC codes are randomly drawn from the electronic hopper. Each UPC owner is required to retain an FDA-specified sample quantity of each production batch for an FDA-specified period of time. The FDA already has similar language in FDA Regulation 21CFR101.9(g). They just need to tighten it up a little.

When the UPC code is drawn from the electronic hopper, a background-checked person goes to the UPC owner's facility and collects a USDA-specified production batch sample of product carrying the UPC code. That batch is equally divided and delivered to two independent companies that do nutrition label testing. The identity of the UPC owner is concealed. The sample batch is tested for PSS (net carb) content. If both independent companies report a PSS count equal to or less than the UPC owner's count, everything is fine. If one independent company reports a PSS (net carb) count of more than the UPC owner's count and one independent company reports a PSS count of equal to or less than the UPC owner's count, everything is still fine. But, if both independent companies report a PSS count of more than the UPC owner's count, the number of understated PSS (net carbs) is averaged and the company who owns the UPC gets to pay into the Freedom Fund for the entire FDA specified production batch.

Using the Victoria labels as an example, the per-serving PSS (net carb) gap between the two labels is five grams. If Victoria didn't have such good quality controls, the label on the newer jar of marinara sauce would understate PSS (net carbs) by five grams per half-cup serving. There are 10 servings of marinara sauce in the jar. That would understate the *container* PSS (net carbs) by 50 grams. The amount of contribution to the Freedom Fund would be short changed by 12.5¢. See how this type of error can add up to lots of money?

To discourage sloppy testing and cheating, this li'l old fat lady recommends charging the UPC owner not one fourth of a penny, but 2¢ for every PSS (net carb) that it has understated on its label. So, the cost of understating the PSS (net carbs) for a jar of marinara sauce would result in the UPC owner paying $1.00 (50 x $0.02) per jar of marinara sauce in that production run. There are no appeals. If the business doesn't pay the amount due within 30 days, they're shut down. If it happens again, the 2¢ for every understated PSS (net carb) doubles to 4¢ to 8¢ to 16¢ and so on.

If big business knows they'll pay big money if they're caught being sloppy or cheating, most won't cheat. There can be no upside for big business. By accurately listing the PSS (net carb) count on every UPC container, the final purchaser pays for the *real* bad boy on the block and the Freedom Fund helps pay for 35 years of scientifically unsound US government nutritional policy. By using 5% of the Freedom Fund for enforcement, we can help assure that big business doesn't cheat. All the money collected from the cheaters goes directly back into the Freedom Fund.

Now, how do we make sure the Freedom Fund gets back to the obese, sick baby boomers? We don't want the Freedom Fund to be drained by huge bloated "administrative" costs. When I say huge, I mean the obscene 17% administrative cost that is associated with our commercial health care system.[41] In comparison, the administrative cost associated with Medicare is 5%.[42] This li'l old fat lady believes we should tie the Freedom Funds to the most recent year's estimated census data. The census already tracks those 65 years old and older. Just add up the Freedom Fund contributions and then divvy out the funds according to the census data.

While many old people are poor people, they usually bring their money with them. They don't often require high-paying jobs. Add in the Freedom Fund contributions and baby boomers could generate good jobs and nice income streams for the hospitals, doctors, pharmaceutical companies, and just about everyone else. Remember the $157 billion ($142 billion + $15 billion) from the Freedom Fund? That's a lot of money. So, the Freedom Fund contributions would help encourage counties and states to put out the welcome mat for us old folks.

And America wants us to stay alive and healthy. If we're both alive *and* healthy, we generate the most income for the least amount of expense. Again, from chapter 7, here are the conclusions from an *American Journal of Public Health* study titled "The Benefits of Risk Factor Prevention in Americans Aged 51 Years and Older." *"Effective [diabetes, hypertension, smoking, and obesity] prevention could substantially improve the health of older Americans, and—despite increases in longevity—such benefits could be achieved with little or no additional lifetime medical spending."*[43]

OK, let's review this li'l old fat lady's list of Freedom Fund benefits. This solution would:

- Allow Americans to have their cake and eat it, too.
- Turn the tide of obesity in America to help us regain our health and freedom.
- Not force a single American to change his or her beliefs or behavior.
- Minimize the time, effort, cost, and conflict of fundamental change.
- Position America as the world innovator and leader in nutritional enlightenment.
- Help improve the economic vitality of America and even increase our export revenues.
- Address the growing financial burden of the exploding obese ill baby boomer population.
- Allow America to play America's game.

Now, when you have fundamental change, not everyone who's winning today will win tomorrow. When fundamental change occurs, there will be both old losers and new winners. But, compared to the 200-million-plus overweight and obese Americans who can become winners, the number of big business losers is very small. So, I'm going to take a moment and speak to some of the old losers and new winners.

OLD LOSERS

Sugar Cane and Sugar Beet Farmers. You are farmers first. Go find something else to grow. Just think *New & Improved!* Jim Simon (board member of the Sugar Association) can't whine about this li'l old fat lady's Freedom Fund Marketing Strategy because it doesn't just "single out one food." Every company who's peddling high PSS obesity, diabetes, heart disease, (and more) foods is in the same boat.

Honey Bee Keepers. You have bees. Although the demand for honey will drop, the demand for bees will explode. All those millions upon millions of acres of *New & Improved!* wheat, corn, rice, and potatoes will need bees for pollination.

Bariatric Surgeons. You are surgeons first. Go find something else to cut on. Better yet, retool your skills and become bariatric *physicians*. Instead of ignoring your .03% surgery death rate, you can brag about your "90%-plus-weight-loss-and-return-to-good-health success rate." (This li'l old fat lady is betting that's what the number would be.)

Pharmaceutical Companies peddling obesity, diabetes, heart disease, hypertension, and other medications that are needed because of the *real* bad boy on the block. These money-making diseases aren't going to disappear overnight or even next year or next decade. So, focus on next quarter's earnings and get your Strategic Marketing folks to figure out how to cash in on *New & Improved!* The Freedom Fund will allow the obese sick baby boomers to be able to continue to buy your expensive "designer" drugs for a long, long time. Ditto for the doctors, hospitals, and medical supply companies.

Coke, Pepsi, and Other Soft Drink Companies. You aren't really losers. Americans are going to continue to drink your sodas. But, you need to be willing to offer more *New & Improved!* low PSS soft drinks instead of the "leaded" stuff you're now peddling. If some Americans want to continue to drink your "leaded" sodas, they should be willing to "carry their own weight."

NEW WINNERS

$62 Billion Weight Loss Industry. There's so much opportunity here it makes my head hurt. But you need to change your business model from peddling false hope to peddling low PSS foods that will enable Americans to once again become slim and healthy. Why? Because the average American can't currently trot down to their local grocery store and buy low PSS foods. You can fill this gap. Private label the low PSS food options that are already available and show your customers how to use them. Teach Americans how to cook and bake using the *New & Improved!* low PSS sweeteners and flours. Help them have their cake and eat it too. They'll love you and pay you handsomely.

Beef, Chicken, Pork, and Dairy Industries. Since the villains are no longer calories, fat, and cholesterol, demand for your products will explode. Instead of the old statement, "go for the gold," Americans will "go for the cheese." Ditto with the saturated fat industry and the nut industry.

Processed Food Industry. This li'l old fat lady is actually handing you a huge gift. Instead of just competing head to head, you now have the golden opportunity to change the rules. Come up with *New & Improved!* delicious, nutritious processed foods, and 311-million-plus Americans will open their wallets. And many of those little low PSS companies who have just been plugging along stand to gain big time. Unfortunately, some of them will be gobbled up by the big boys so that they can accelerate the introduction of their *New & Improved!* processed food options.

Processed Food Nutrition Testing Industry. Get ready to hire.

Fast Food Industry. Now that nobody's on a diet anymore, you'll see your revenues soar. The trick is to make your *New & Improved!* menu look, taste, and smell just like your old high PSS obesity-, diabetes-, and heart-disease-causing menu. Again, here is a cardinal rule this li'l old fat lady learned from the school-of-hard-knocks. The more you can make your *New & Improved!* menu look, taste, smell, feel, sound, and act like what folks are already accustomed to, the better.

Corn, Wheat, Rice, and Potato Industries. Just like "designer label" coffee beans, you can now peddle high protein, low carbohydrate, "designer label" versions of your commodity. You can make more money with your *New & Improved!* product because it offers the consumer something he or she will value and be willing to pay more for. "Normal weight and healthy" is the most compelling marketing message in the world.

Agricultural Equipment and Supply Industry. When the wheat, corn, rice, and potato farmers figure out that they can cash in on *New & Improved!* they're going to need more of what you peddle.

Transportation Industry. Just think. All that *New & Improved!* wheat, corn, rice, and potatoes will need to be moved from the field to somewhere else.

***New & Improved!* Fruit and Vegetable Industries.** The sky is the limit.

200-Million-Plus Overweight and Obese Americans. No more dieting! You *can* have your cake and eat it too!

CHAPTER 11

Let Freedom Ring—Again

Human beings, who are almost unique in having the ability to learn from the experience of others, are also remarkable for their apparent disinclination to do so.—Douglas Adams (1952–2001)

Editorial by Dana Carpender, CarbSmart Managing Editor,
www.CarbSmart.com

Posted June 19, 2011
Sandy Lee writes:

I just can't understand why the powers that be can't restudy, re-view and re-evaluate such nonsense!! Why won't main stream just turn around and say YES the obesity problem is due to SUGARS and such useless carbs Period!

Granted, there is now a push to get rid of corn syrups in everything and a push toward more fiber/whole grains and no trans fats, all great steps, but just rip that old band aid off and face up to the Whole Truth??? NOW

Sandy, I wish it were that easy. There are a whole lot of obstacles for us to get around.

First of all, there are no monolithic Powers That Be. There are a whole lot of different Powers That Be, and they all make up their minds separately, in their own time, and they all have their own motives. There are, for instance, medical schools, a whole lot of medical schools, and a great deal of the funding for those medical schools comes from the pharmaceutical industry, as does a lot of the money for medical research. That's a clear danger, but the alternative, at least as far as I can tell, is to fund medical schools and medical research with tax money. For good or ill, a large faction of Americans is very much against that.

There are government agencies like the USDA and the FDA, who, again, are deeply beholden to various industries. There are professional associations like the AHA and the ADA, ditto.

There are all the individual doctors, some of whom are savvy to low carb, some of whom are just starting to glimpse the value of carb restriction because of positive reports from their patients, and some of them who are deeply resistant to the whole concept. Why the resistance, when it appears so obvious to all of us that carb restriction works? First of all, it goes against everything they've been taught. But perhaps more powerful, imagine how it must feel to be a doctor who has, for thirty years, in good faith, recommended a low fat, low cholesterol diet, the substitution of animal fats with vegetable oils, all of the conventional wisdom of the past few decades, to your patients, only to face the creeping realization that not only may you not have helped, you may be responsible for hundreds, if not thousands, of cases of obesity, heart disease, diabetes, infertility, and even cancer. How very human to deny, deny, deny, not simply to one's patients, but to one's self.

Let's not forget, too, that all of those doctors are people first, with their own food addictions, and their own emotions. Emotion is a big part of this. People are very attached to the idea of food as love, and it is painful for them to realize that Grandma baking them cookies, Mom making them a birthday cake, the junk food they associate with summer days at the beach, all of that, is dangerous. It hurts. It's like admitting that the relationship with the guy you adore just isn't working out, and never will. That's true for doctors as much as for everyone else.

Another branch of the Powers That Be is the registered dieticians; they face the same stuff the doctors do, with the additional burden of nearly always having to administer the diets the doctors recommend, regardless of their own understanding. Even the RDs who accept that low carb diets work can lose their jobs if they recommend such a diet against doctor's orders.

Then there's the mainstream media, everybody's favorite whipping boy. Yes, they embraced low carb in 2003, because it was NEW and EXCITING and CONTROVERSIAL, and gee, who knew you could lose weight eating steak instead of pasta salad? But, of course, the media as a whole has the attention span of a hyperactive five year old who has drunk an entire pitcher of Kool Aid. As soon as low carb was becoming generally accepted, it had to be dead, because they needed to move on to the Next Big Thing, and the fact that the human body doesn't change every year be damned.

More importantly, the mainstream media, and especially television and the women's magazines, is funded by advertising. What kind of advertising? You tell me: What percentage of the ads you see on TV are for processed food, fast food or chain restaurants, or drugs, both over-the-counter and prescription? How many ads do you see for low carb commodities like steak and salad greens? There's no ad revenue in low carb. That means there's little incentive for the media to report the good news.

Which leads to our biggest obstacle: The vast fraction of our economy that is built on bad diet and its consequences. What would happen to the economy -- I mean, really think about this -- what would happen if overnight everyone stopped swilling down soda, eating piles of sugary, starchy junk? What would happen to the restaurant industry, the food processing industry, the agricultural industry, the pharmaceutical industry, heck, the dental treatment industry? Even things like the cosmetics industry would take a hit, because people who eat right naturally have better skin and hair than people who don't. There are very powerful economic forces that have every reason to want the status quo to continue. Addiction and ill-health are very, very lucrative.

In short, "the Powers That Be" pretty much amounts to the whole dang society. There is no short cut. It's a matter of reaching people one at a time, of telling our stories, of speaking out, of saying to the doctor "yes, I've lost weight and my blood work is better -- it's because I'm on Atkins," of telling our friends, "I know, I ate a low fat diet too, but it just made my diabetes worse; let me tell you what helped." It's like Gandhi said: You must be the change you want to see in the world.

Of course, Gandhi also said, "First they ignore you, then they ridicule you, then they fight you, then you win."

I'm pleased to report that we're way past the "ignore" phase, moving from the "ridicule" into the "fight" stage. I hope to see "win" in my lifetime.

© 2004, 2011 by Dana Carpender. Used by permission of the author.

Dana Carpender, managing editor of CarbSmart (*www.CarbSmart.com*), nails the issues right on the head. And yes, we *are* in the "fight" stage. Here are some examples of the "fight." On June 1, 2012, the AP headline stated, *"NYC proposes ban on large sodas at restaurants."*

> In his latest effort to fight obesity in this era of Big Gulps and triple bacon cheeseburgers, Mayor Michael Bloomberg is proposing an unprecedented ban on large servings of soda and other sugary drinks at restaurants, delis, sports arenas and movie theaters….At a Burger King in Manhattan, retired postal worker Bobby Brown didn't like the mayor's ideas, saying people should be "free to choose what they drink or eat." But Joseph Alan, a chauffeur eating at a nearby Subway, said his overweight friends' eating habits ultimately affect him, too. "I tell them. This is affecting our insurance, because charges go up more treating people with diabetes and other health problems. I don't want to pay more for health insurance so people can have these drinks!"[1]

And, on April 1, 2012, CBS's *60 Minutes* featured Dr. Robert Lustig, MD, a pediatric endocrinologist at the University of California. (The video is at *www.cbsnews.com/sections/60minutes/main3415.shtml.* Type "toxic sugar" into the search box. You will be astonished to learn that our doctors and scientists are saying that sugar not only causes obesity, but is also extremely addictive, and is used by some cancers to grow.) This is what CBS News had to say:

> Dr. Lustig treats sick, obese children, who he believes are primarily sick because of the amount of sugar they ingest. He says that this sugar not only leads to obesity, but to "Type 2 diabetes, hypertension and heart disease itself." Something needs to be done says Dr. Lustig. "Ultimately, this is a public health crisis…you have to do big things and you have to do them across the board," he tells [Dr. Sanjay] Gupta. "Tobacco and alcohol are perfect examples," he says, referring to the regulations imposed on their consumption and the warnings on their labels. "I think sugar belongs in this exact same wastebasket."[2]

This li'l old fat lady agrees with Mayor Bloomberg's "fight" and Dr. Lustig's "fight" but believes neither "fight" goes far enough. Eliminating excess sugar will help but will *not* solve the obesity epidemic in this country. Sugar is just one form of carbohydrates, and there are excessive carbohydrates in just about every bottle, jar, box, can, and bag that consumers put into their grocery carts. This li'l old fat lady applauds Dr. Lustig's statement, "You have to do big things, and you have to do them across the board." But we need to be focused on PSS—on the entire *real* bad boy on the block—not on just chopping him off at the knees. To repeat Dr. Lustig, "You have to do big things, and you have to do them across the board."

However, instead of focusing on "fight," this li'l old fat lady's Freedom Fund Marketing Strategies focus on "win." They focus on trying to get *the vast fraction of our economy that is built on bad diet and its consequences* to turn the kaleidoscope to see how many businesses can make more money. These Freedom Fund Marketing Strategies allow Americans to have their cake and eat it too. They don't require a single American to change his or her behavior or beliefs. And they offer a solution that could help minimize the financial strain that baby boomers are placing on our country. But, because these strategies do involve fundamental change, there will still be lots of individuals and big businesses that will engage in the "cast doubt" and "fundamental-change-hysterical-fear" routines. That's just the way we humans are.

As this li'l old fat lady contemplated sitting down to write this book, I hesitated and procrastinated. I lacked the courage to write down what I had learned from my 90-pound weight loss and return-to-good-health journey during the past eight years. Why? Because, although I was certain that my knowledge would be of value to many others, I was just as certain that there would be lots of doubters and naysayers. I knew there would be those from big government, big business, and even consumers who would attack this book even though the scientific, medical, and government research is absolutely pristine. I would be attacked even though the attackers would offer no real solutions of their own.

As I was hesitating, the September 11, 2001 World Trade Center disaster's 10-year anniversary memorial services began. I watched hours and hours of television coverage. I watched as the families of those lost expressed their terrible anguish and pain at losing their loved ones. I saw some of the majestic, unselfish heroism that took place during this national tragedy. We Americans must always remember and never forget September 11, 2001.

During the television coverage, a message kept appearing on the TV screen. It was, "What Will YOU Do?" What will *you* do to remember? It took several days and many repeats of that message during the September 11, 2011, anniversary memorial services, but I finally realized what I could do. I could write this book for America. I could risk being attacked and labeled a fraud like Dr. Robert C. Atkins was almost 40 years ago. I could risk what I call the "Smith Thammasaroj phenomenum."[3]

You know who he is, of course. The whole world must know who Smith Thammasaroj is. Well, if you, like many others, don't, he's the fellow who tried to prevent the deaths of 227,898[4] innocent humans in 13 countries.[5] Yes, it was the December 26, 2004, Asian tsunami disaster. I realize that these humans weren't Americans, but they were still humans. Each one of them had a right to live. And almost every one of them had loved ones who experienced horrible anguish and pain. Without minimizing the horrific tragedy of September 11, 2001, in America, just realize that the loss of life on December 26, 2004, was approximately 67 times greater than what happened here in America. Try to envision 67 World Trade Center disasters. It is truly beyond comprehension.

Here's a little background information on this tragic event. According to *The Nation*, Bangkok's independent newspaper, "In September 1998, Smith [Thammasaroj], then serving his stint at the Communications Ministry, wrote a letter of complaint to Jadet In-sawarng, the governor of Phuket, who threatened to assault Smith because his tsunami talk had been causing panic within the tourism and real estate [big business] industries. The media tended to disregard Smith's warnings, and even mocked him. Od Turbo, a columnist for Thai Rath newspaper, assured readers that they should not panic, saying there would surely be warnings and predictions if any natural disasters were about to occur."[6]

And, according to the East Asian Pastoral Institute: "Human safety was also sacrificed on the altar of tourist interests [big business] in Thailand in the last decade. Smith Thammasaroj—formerly the head of Thailand's meteorological office—was forced to resign under a cloud in 1998. He was accused of scaremongering when he warned that the south-west coast faced a deadly tsunami. The tourist industry [big business] accused him of jeopardizing the industry by scaring away foreign tourists from areas around the island of Phuket. If his warnings had been taken seriously and monitoring equipment had been put in place, many of the 9,000 [Thailand only—the total death toll was 227,898] who are dead or missing could have been saved. One week after the tsunami the Prime Minister of Thailand, Thaksin Schinawatra, appointed [Smith] Thammasaroj as a minister in charge of the newly established national disaster warning office."[7] Yes, hindsight is 20/20.

The greatest tragedy of the Asian tsunami disaster is that Smith Thammasaroj spoke up but no one would listen until it was too late. It's a perfect example of Douglas Adam's statement, *Human beings, who are almost unique in having the ability to learn from the experience of others, are also remarkable for their apparent disinclination to do so.* Immediately after the deadly tsunami, Thammasaroj was quoted as saying, "Now I can die in peace because what I warned has come true. Still, I feel sorry that I could not help save the lives of thousands of people."[8] But maybe it is possible that Smith's very sad statement might not have to be completely true.

Perhaps we Americans can learn from this terrible tragedy. Perhaps Smith Thammasaroj's example can help us Americans avoid our own looming disaster. It's the deadly obesity tsunami caused by 35 years of scientifically unsound US government nutritional policy. While the obesity epidemic in America will not produce the same horrific, 227,898 lives lost in a single event, it will prematurely claim many more Americans in a slow motion tragic drama over the next few decades. Most obese people don't just die peacefully in their sleep. The associated human suffering and medical costs are staggering.

Perhaps we Americans should listen a little less to Weight Watchers' glamorous Jennifer Hudson sing, "Because It Works" and a little more to the medical doctors, scientists, dietitians, and nutritional expert authors. We're not talking Snake Oil Salesmen. Many of them have pedigrees a mile long—here's just one example. Dr. Stephen D. Phinney, MD, PhD, is a physician-scientist who has spent 35 years studying diet, exercise, fatty acids, and inflammation, has published over 70 papers, and holds several patents. He received his MD from Stanford University, his PhD in nutritional biochemistry from the Massachusetts Institute of Technology (MIT), and postdoctoral training at the University of Vermont and Harvard.[9] Along with Jeff S. Volek, PhD, RD, he's the coauthor of *The Art and Science of Low Carbohydrate Living* and *The Art and Science of Low Carbohydrate Performance* for athletes. These two physician-scientists, along with Eric C. Westman, MD, are also coauthors of *The New Atkins for a New You.*

In addition, there are the voices of Richard Bernstein, MD; Jonny Bowden, PhD; Dana Carpender; Andrew DiMino; Mary Dan Eades, MD; Michael R. Eades, MD; Andreas Eenfeldt, MD; Jacqueline Eberstein, RN; Richard Feinman, PhD; Michael D. Fox, MD; Dr. Eric H. Kossoff, MD; Robert Lustig, MD; Jimmy Moore; Barry Sears, PhD; Gary Taubes; Mary Vernon, MD; Terry Wahls, MD; Jay Wortman, MD; and countless others. They're all saying pretty much the same thing, but America hasn't been listening. No—many of us continue to stubbornly cling to the old, outdated dietary dogma that has caused this tragic situation. But just maybe it *is* time we started listening so that many Americans will still have a chance to run from the deadly obesity tsunami that has been caused by 35 years of scientifically unsound US government nutritional policy.

This li'l old fat lady also believes America needs to accept the fact that we currently have too many obese, sick baby boomers. If we 78 million baby boomers don't want to end up being denied medical care and continuing to have our Social Security benefits chiseled away, we need to speak up as Americans and demand accountability for 35 years of scientifically unsound US government nutritional policy. We need to realize that it's the baby boomers who have been harmed the most, because it can take 35 years for the *real* bad boy to rear his ugly head. Remember, the 20- to 30-year-olds in 1977 have now become the 55- to 65-year-olds in 2012.

It's *not* just because we baby boomers are getting old. If someone pulls this "cast doubt" routine, point out the 2004 *American Journal of Clinical Nutrition* study titled "Increased consumption of refined carbohydrates and the epidemic of type 2 diabetes in the United States: an ecological assessment."[10] Then point out our federal government's NIH (National Institute of Health) website.[11] As of 2008, the rates of diabetes for those over 65 years old is over 700% higher than for those younger than 44 years old. For diabetes patients, their human suffering is horrific, and health care costs are much higher. This information is located in chapter 3, "The *Real* Bad Boy On The Block." Just go back and take a quick look at the scientific research numbers and charts—they tell a very powerful story. Then there's the smoking gun from the correlation between obesity, Alzheimer's, metastasized cancer, and…the list just goes on and on.

Diagnosed and Undiagnosed Diabetes

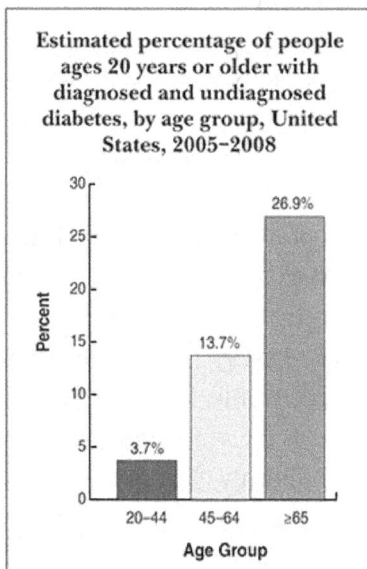

Estimated percentage of people ages 20 years or older with diagnosed and undiagnosed diabetes, by age group, United States, 2005–2008

Source: 2005–2008 National Health and Nutrition Examination Survey[12]

Here's what 35 years of scientifically unsound US government nutritional policy means for older Americans. By age 65, around two-thirds of all seniors have at least one chronic disease and see seven physicians. Twenty percent of those older than 65 have five or more chronic diseases, see 14 physicians—and average 40 doctor visits a year.[13] Medicare does *not* cover all these costs. With the monthly premiums, deductibles, co-pays, and doughnut holes (a huge gap in prescription medicine coverage), many obese, sick baby boomers are seeing their retirement days become poverty days. There are too many cases where baby boomers are being forced to choose between an empty refrigerator and expensive prescription medicine that is required due to decades of excessive carbohydrate consumption.

And the cost of Medicare just keeps increasing. Here's what the AP says in an article with the headline *Medicare costs to reduce Social Security increase*: "That didn't last long. About 55 million Social Security recipients will get their first increase in benefits next year since 2009—a 3.5% raise. But higher Medicare premiums could erase part of it… AARP Executive Vice President Nancy LeaMond is quoted as saying, 'Medicare premiums are also expected to rise for many. And with the decline in housing values, deep losses to retirement and savings accounts, and skyrocketing health and prescription drug costs, millions of older Americans continue to struggle to make ends meet.' "[14] Yes, it *is* the baby boomers who have been harmed the most by 35 years of scientifically unsound US government nutritional policy.

This li'l old fat lady thinks that the AARP should do a little less in the way of holding out a donation hat and a little more in the way of holding out a nice stout stick. As Fred Griesbach, AARP Campaigns, says, "The next President and Congress may well determine the future of Medicare and Social Security. Don't let Washington make decisions about your future without hearing from you."[15] It's up to each and every one of us baby boomers to make our voices heard. With 78 million of us, just maybe the politicians might be interested in what we have to say.

We need to say enough is enough. We need to say we believe that 35 years of scientifically unsound US government nutritional policy has harmed baby boomers the most and that all Americans need to help correct this tragic situation. We *cannot* go back, but we *can* go forward. By putting a tiny price on the head of the *real* bad boy on the block, we can help America take care of our exploding population of obese, sick baby boomers. That tiny price can also help turn the tide of obesity, diabetes, heart disease, and more. Author Malcolm Gladwell calls this a lever, or "The Tipping Point."

"The Tipping Point" of one fourth of a penny will help turn the tide of economic decline that is robbing our citizens of the American Dream. One fourth of a penny can help us turn the kaleidoscope so that big business will realize that it can make more money by developing more nutritious, high protein, low carbohydrate wheat, corn, potato, and rice crops. By doing so, we can leverage our 309,607,601[16] acres of valuable American harvested cropland to produce higher priced, protein rich, low carbohydrate food for Americans as well as generate desperately needed export revenues.

Big business can't "offshore" our American farmland, so we could even begin to turn the tide of poverty that exists in our rural heartland. By offering our citizens more nourishing processed foods that don't cause obesity, diabetes, heart disease, and more, both big business and the average American can win. But, we need to turn the kaleidoscope to see that we can make *Grown in America* a source of national pride. We need to move beyond the low-price-commodity mentality to see that we can actually change the game. Here's an example of this mentality. It's from the National Corn Growers Association's website.

The Low Cost of Corn in Food

Food	Quantity of Corn	Cost ($7/bushel)
Corn Flakes Cereal	12.9 oz in an 18-ounce box	10 cents
Soda/Soft Drink	15 oz wt (as HFCS) in a 2-liter bottle	12 cents
Beef	2.6 lb for 1 lb of beef	33 cents
Pork	3.6 lb for 1 lb of pork	45 cents
Chicken/Turkey	2.6 lb for 1 lb chicken or turkey	33 cents
Eggs	4 lb for 1 doz eggs	42 cents
Milk	1.8 lb for 1 gallon	23 cents

NCGA

Sources: USDA, Beef Checkoff, Pork Board,
National Turkey Federation, American Egg Board

17

Instead of focusing on the essential amino acids in proteins and the essential fatty acids in fats, we focus on the "Low Cost of Corn in Food" and miss the big picture of out-of-control obesity and ill health in this country and the rest of the world. Lots of research has been done to increase crop yields and combat crop diseases, but very little research has been done to improve the nutritional quality.

Even in India, nutritional quality is not a priority. In reference to the high protein, low carbohydrate rice that's being developed, according to University of Agricultural Sciences (UAS) Vice Chancellor K. Narayana Gouda, "Transfer of technology could take time. There aren't enough officials to do this work. At the hobli [cluster of villages] level it is difficult even to get two officials. The university cannot take responsibility as we are already training, researching, and doing technology transfer to a small extent."[18] So it's not just America that's missing the big picture.

This li'l old fat lady believes that when folks need to climb 14,000-foot mountain peaks to avoid becoming obese and ill, our mainstream American foods need to change. Here's the reality. If we don't step up to the plate on the front end, most of us Americans (68.5% and still rising) are going to suffer the consequences on the back end. We're either going to pay up front or down the line. Right now we're paying down the line. Even our 164.6 million precious family member dogs and cats are paying down the line.

We also need to accept that the days of Henry Ford and the Industrial Revolution that made America so rich and powerful are gone. Because "every man is the creature of the age in which he lives," most of us don't realize that before the Industrial Revolution, work was something you did, not someplace you went. America's golden age of sending a man to the moon and launching the Space Shuttle is now behind us. The trade deficit with China—$295 billion in 2011[19]—has eliminated or displaced 2.8 million US jobs between 2001 and 2010.[20] Even our heady days of the computer and information age in America are beginning to wane because so much of the production work can now be "offshored" to other countries where labor costs are much lower.

But, all 7 billion people who inhabit Mother Earth must eat to live, and, across the globe, the rates of obesity continue to rise along with the population. And, over time, those 7 billion people will likely become 8 billion or more. While grass-fed organic chicken, beef, and pork are premium sources of essential protein and essential fats, that option is probably not feasible for all 7 billion people. The majority of humans on this planet will most likely continue to be dependent on things like wheat, corn, rice, and potatoes just for survival. And the obesity rates around the world will continue to rise. So, this li'l old fat lady thinks it's time to change the rules. *It's time for America to play its game.*

Here's how. By leveraging our world-class factor condition of 309,607,601 acres of fertile, American-harvested cropland, we can produce more valuable, high protein, low carbohydrate foods for Americans as well as the rest of the world. America could actually move toward a revitalization of our economy. Remember what coach Herb Brooks kept saying during the final minutes of the historic February 20, 1980, Winter Olympics ice hockey game. His words to his team were, "Play your game. Play your game. Play your game. Play your game."

America's game is Innovation. We're the nation who mainstreamed the automobile, airplane, and computer. The Internet started in America, and we played a critical role in making the lightbulb and telephone ubiquitous around the world. We even put the first man on the moon. And there are countless other examples of America's innovations. So, going forward, *we could position America as the new world leader in nutritional enlightenment and innovation.* America knows how to produce the best *New & Improved!* foods for our citizens and the rest of the world. Once again, we're the world leaders in Innovation!

Here's how we can play our game that's based on innovation. If we develop more valuable, high protein, low carbohydrate crops, our exports will increase. Here's the headline again: *Export markets paying premiums for high protein wheat.*[21] With a little old-fashioned American ingenuity, we could produce more high protein wheat, as well as high protein corn, potatoes, rice, and more. We could move commodity grains out of the 1960s "canned coffee" pricing model into today's Starbucks "designer label" pricing model. Yes, a 21st century agricultural gold rush could actually occur in America. With an Internet-enabled explosion of viable small farm businesses offering *New & Improved!* micro-brewery–type, specialty, low carbohydrate, high protein grain products and good old-fashioned customer service, the economic picture in this country could improve dramatically.

Here's where we are now regarding farms in America. After decades of financial decline, most farms are small (54.4% are less than 99 acres and 31% are less than 500 acres). The annual sales generated by these farms are miniscule (annually 59.8% generate less than $10,000 and 18.3% generate less than $50,000). And the vast majority of farms are owned by 1,906,335 individuals (86.5%) rather than big corporations.[22] So yes, with higher priced more nutritious "designer label" agricultural crops, the small farm economic dynamics could improve dramatically.

Then there's the pioneering innovation of a company called Generation UCAN.[23] Generation UCAN offers sports drinks for athletes, and they've figured out how to tweak carbohydrates so that they will become a low PSS. This li'l old fat lady believes that if Generation UCAN can, other American companies can, too.

Here's what Generation UCAN has done. Using "leaded" non-GMO cornstarch, they've developed patent pending "SuperStarch." Below is a graph that shows the difference in insulin response from their "unleaded" product versus typical insulin response from "leaded" carbohydrates. The top line is maltodextrin (a sugar in sheep's clothing). The bottom line is SuperStarch. As you can see below, the insulin response from consuming maltodextrin was nearly eight times greater than that from consuming SuperStarch.[24] *The top line represents what we're doing to our poor overworked pancreas every time we consume "leaded" carbohydrates. The bottom line represents the ideal in dietary strategy.*

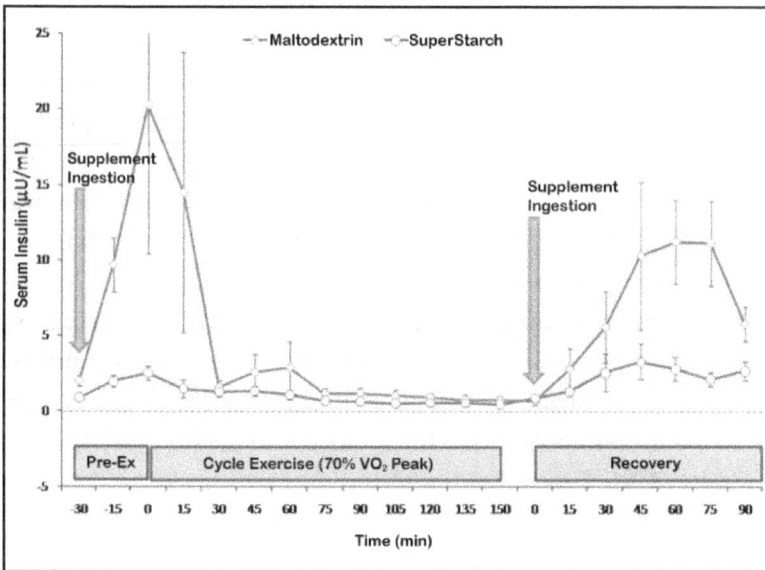

25

How do we know this is graph is true? Generation UCAN states that these results are from a carefully controlled, double blinded experiment conducted at the University of Oklahoma via an independent IRB (Institutional Review Board) process.[26] What is an IRB? An IRB is an appropriately constituted group that has been formally designated to review and monitor biomedical research involving human subjects.[27] IRBs are responsible for critical oversight functions for research conducted on human subjects to ensure that the research is "scientific," "ethical," and "regulatory."[28] So the IRB makes sure the humans are not harmed, but it doesn't look at the research results to see if they are actually true. Although this li'l old fat lady is confident that the folks who conducted the research at the University of Oklahoma are ethical and documented the truth, there's currently no mechanism in place to assure consumers that we're not dealing with Snake Oil Salesmen.

Americans need to be confident that we're not dealing with Snake Oil Salesmen. We need the equivalent of the UL mark that stands for Underwriters Laboratory. UL was founded back in 1894 by William Henry Merrill under the name Underwriters' Electrical Bureau, the Electrical Bureau of the National Board of Fire Underwriters. The bureau's first test was conducted on March 24, 1894, on noncombustible insulation materials for "Mr. Shields."[29] The UL mark on a product means that UL has tested and evaluated representative samples of that product and determined that they meet UL requirements.[30] Today, there are dozens of UL marks made for Asia, Europe, Latin America, and North America.[31] In 2011, 22.4 billion UL marks appeared on products made by 67,798 manufacturers around the globe.[32]

Because food nutrition rules are changing, we need to implement the same UL-caliber quality certification for our foods. Here's why. Today, carbohydrates typically cause the pancreas to emit insulin. But, with the pioneering work of companies like Generation UCAN, this rule is changing. In the future, more and more carbohydrates will become "unleaded" and cause minimal insulin response. But, there's currently no way to know which carbohydrates are "unleaded." And, according to diabetes expert Richard K. Bernstein, MD, some foods that say they have few or zero carbs actually cause a significant insulin response in humans.[33] So it's time to change the rules. To make sure we Americans are not dealing with Snake Oil Salesmen, this li'l old fat lady has designed a new logo that could be used to certify that the foods consumers buy are truly a low PSS. Here's the new *lowPSS* SM logo.

And here's the Marketing Concept. Foods that have this logo would undergo a stringent certification process that scientifically measures the food against a standard. In the graph above, Generation's UCAN SuperStarch was measured against maltodextrin (a sugar in sheep's clothing). So Generation UCAN's product, while containing lots of carbohydrates, could actually qualify as a low PSS (Pancreas Stimulating Substance). This high carbohydrate food didn't cause a large insulin response! It's a huge innovation and Generation UCAN might just become the first company to sport the new *lowPSS* SM logo.

So yes, between *New & Improved!* corn, wheat, rice, and potatoes, and "unleaded" innovations from companies like Generation UCAN, this li'l old fat lady believes that

America has what it takes to turn our *Titanic* around. But we need to think outside the box to be able to turn the kaleidoscope to see what *can* be rather than what *is*. Just maybe this *is* a good time to change the rules. Once more, by changing the rules, we can:

- Allow Americans to have their cake and eat it too.

- Turn the tide of obesity in America to help us regain our health and freedom.

- Not force a single American to change his or her beliefs or behavior.

- Minimize the time, effort, cost, and conflict of fundamental change.

- Position America as the world innovator and leader in nutritional enlightenment.

- Help improve the economic vitality of America and even increase our export revenues.

- Address the growing financial burden of the exploding population of obese, ill baby boomers.

- Allow America to play America's game.

Now, back to us overweight and obese folks. What this li'l old fat lady is really suggesting is that we overweight and obese Americans stop beating our heads against the wall. For too many decades our federal government has been telling us it's all our fault. If we fat folks wouldn't be weak-willed wimps and biggie-size everything at the fast food joints, we would become lean and healthy. Even now, the USDA continues to tell us we just need to count calories and exercise more. If we will just eat more fruits, vegetables, whole grains, and less Phat!, we will find the Holy Grail.

For the past 35 years, this scientifically unsound nutritional strategy hasn't worked. During this time, all America has done is become fatter and fatter and unhealthier and unhealthier. In far too many counties in America, we're seeing the life expectancy fail to rise or we're seeing it actually drop. To repeat Einstein one more time, *"The definition of insanity is doing the same thing over and over again and expecting different results."* Our current diet doctrine of counting calories and restricting fats is insane, and it's time for a change.

What this li'l old fat lady is really suggesting is that we stop asking Americans to defy Mother Nature. Instead, we need to fundamentally improve the nutritional quality of our foods and find new outside-the-box ways to encourage our citizens to seek out physical activity. Let's figure out how to work *with* Mother Nature, not against her.

We also need to realize that, like the cause of yellow fever description at the beginning of this book, our understanding of nutrition will continue to change over time. Using yellow fever as an analogy, we now understand that mosquitoes cause yellow fever, but don't yet know that "there are three epidemiologically different infectious cycles" called urban, sylvatic, and savannah.

Like the yellow fever and mosquito example, we are just beginning to understand that excessive carbohydrate consumption is the real culprit. But we don't yet know exactly why. Soon, this li'l old fat lady's explanations will become outdated. Soon, we will have a better understanding of why some folks struggle so much with their weight while others suffer the consequences of excessive carbohydrate consumption in more subtle, insidious ways.

One intriguing clue is the role that our body's mitochondria may play in the obesity drama and other diseases like multiple sclerosis and epilepsy. Mitochondria are the little sausage-shaped organelles inside the cells that convert the energy stored in food to ATP, the energy currency of the body.[34]

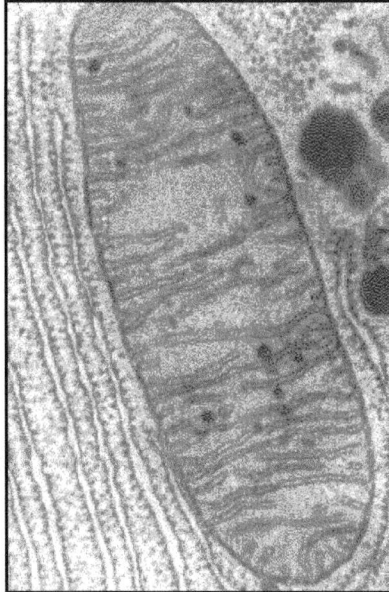

Regarding mitochondria and obesity, the new book, *The Art and Science of Low Carbohydrate Living*, by Jeff S. Volek, PhD, RD, and Stephen D. Phinney, MD, PhD, states, "To facilitate fat utilization, muscle triglycerides in trained individuals [athletes] are localized near mitochondria within cells. In obesity, the muscle triglyceride pool is more inert and tends to be stored in droplets away from mitochondria. There is also a decreased number and size of mitochondria and overall reduced oxidative capacity in the untrained obese person."[35] Although we don't yet fully understand how or why, there may be a link between our mitochondria and obesity.

Then there's Dr. Terry Wahls MD, a physician who was struck down by a relentlessly progressive neurodegenerative disorder. It's called MS, or multiple sclerosis. By nutritionally focusing on the mitochondria that is in our cells, Dr. Wahls was able to regain her freedom to sit, walk, ride a bike, and do other physical activities. While this li'l old fat lady doesn't eat quite as well as Dr. Wahls, I believe her strategies represent the direction we should all be going regarding human nutrition. I strongly encourage you to watch her 17-minute YouTube video.[36] I know it's long, but watching it is definitely worth your time.

Next, there is Dr. Eric H. Kossoff, MD, a specialist in neurologic disorders. He uses a ketogenic (low carbohydrate) diet as a treatment for epilepsy seizures. "Studies from all over the world have consistently shown that, when used as the first treatment, about 60% of children will have at least a 50% reduction in their seizures within 6 months…. For decades, ketones were seen as acting like a drug, with their elevated levels being the sole reason this diet worked. However, researchers now believe the diet has favorable effects on your mitochondria (energy producing parts of your brain cells), which may be due to the high fat intake, stabilized blood glucose, or increased brain chemicals called neurotransmitters which can suppress seizures."[37]

The brain is still a great mystery and we will continue to expand our knowledge of the role our brain plays in our physical health. This li'l old fat lady has noticed a consistent theme, in almost every book referenced, of the negative role that stress plays in weight loss. In other words, increased stress correlates with increased weight or inability to lose weight. As this book neared completion, this li'l old fat lady's stress levels soared. So did my weight. While it was just a few pounds compared to the 90 pounds lost, the only variable that had changed was my stress. So, here's a curious observation.

This li'l old fat lady can remember the 1960s, an era of hippies who practiced something called Transcendental Meditation. Back then, most folks just thought they were nuts. But, fifty years later, big TV names like Dr. Oz and Oprah Winfrey are now speaking out about the benefits of TM. Even my physician, Dr. Leder, is convinced that meditation can improve our physical health. Is it possible that TM is also a fundamental change? Is it possible that those psychedelic hippies weren't as dumb as we thought? What might happen if we paired up TM with the latest science on Low Carbohydrate High Fat nutrition? Today, there are no answers, but tomorrow may bring new understanding.

Thanks to the Internet, our ability to access information and communicate with one another has dramatically improved in recent years. Without the Internet, the scientific research and government publications referenced in this book would have been out of reach of this li'l old fat lady. Just a few years ago, this book would not have been self-published and available on Amazon.com. A few years ago, this book would not have been written. Before self-publishing and Internet marketing came of age, nutritional expert authors were subjected to censorship by mainstream publishers and editors. And only a few mainstream nutritional books were stocked in the bricks-and-mortar bookstores. Here's what nutritional expert Michael R. Eades, MD, says on his blog.

> In my opinion, *The Art and Science of Low Carbohydrate Living* [self-published] is simply the best how-to book on low-carb dieting ever written. As I wrote above, it is the book I wish MD [Mary Dan Eades, MD] and I had written. The reason we didn't write it is because a) some of this information wasn't available when we last wrote a book (much of it is now available thanks to the work of Drs. Volek and Phinney), and b) no mainstream publisher would pay an author for this book. If a mainstream publisher would buy it, the editor would force the authors to change it.[38]

Speaking of excellent blogs, you really should check out *www.DietDoctor.com*, a website hosted by Andreas Eenfeldt, MD. Dr. Eenfeldt's home is Sweden, where low-carb is also becoming mainstream. I know I mentioned Dr. Eenfeldt's website back in chapter 6, but it's worth mentioning again. This website has got all sorts of valuable information that can help you regain your freedom and health. Dr. Eenfeldt features Dr. Robert Lustig, MD, the pediatrician who says that "sugar not only leads to obesity, but to type 2 diabetes, hypertension and heart disease itself."[39] If you want a crystal clear primer on the *real* bad boy on the block, type the following URL into your browser: http://www.dietdoctor.com/?s=lustig and scroll down until you get to *The Skinny on Obesity* episode number one. You're looking for a picture of a fat man with the words "Metabolic Syndrome" and eight little circles with the words *diabetes*, *heart disease*, *hypertension*, *dementia*, *cancer*, etc. Episodes two through four are just as enlightening.

This is what the low-carb medical and scientific experts keep trying to tell us. Just like Smith Thammasaroj, the experts understand that, before the devastating tsunami wave, the water first goes out, leaving an empty beach. Obesity is that empty beach. The low-carb medical and scientific experts are telling us where to run, but too many of us are not listening. We're still listening to Weight Watchers' glamorous Jennifer Hudson sing, "Because It Works."

As I've stated before, some of these li'l old fat lady's explanations will soon become outdated. So, it's OK if folks argue with me about some of my conclusions. And it's OK if folks want to argue about my Freedom Fund Marketing Strategies. But, no one can argue that this li'l old fat lady has managed to do something that 98.4% of folks fail to do—lose 90 pounds and not regain it all and more. As a bonus, I've also managed to regain my health and personal freedom—and I did it without dieting. I did it by defying current USDA diet doctrine. As a result, I have my cake and eat it too. You too can have your cake and eat it too.

This li'l old fat lady hopes that more and more Americans will get fed up like I did. But until this happens, big business and big government will continue to conduct business as usual, because we're the consumers and we're in charge. One fourth of a penny is a small price to pay for America's freedom. Even if you don't want to believe that decades of excessive carbohydrate consumption has caused the tragic obesity, diabetes, and heart disease outcomes in America, the price to turn the tide is only one fourth of a penny. But, if we wait to react until the giant obesity tsunami wave is directly overhead, it will be too late for many of us.

I'm just one li'l old fat lady. In most ways I'm just like the other 200-million-plus overweight and obese Americans out there. I hope there are a few who will be able to learn from my experience. I hope there will be a few Americans who will be able to turn the kaleidoscope and raise themselves above the ideas of the time. It would be truly American to prove Douglas Adams wrong when he said, "*Human beings, who are almost unique in having the ability to learn from the experience of others, are also remarkable for their apparent disinclination to do so.*"

There's a 2009 book and movie titled *The Help*, written by Kathryn Stockett. It's a captivating story about racial bigotry during 1962 in Jackson, Mississippi. While racial bigotry and obesity may not initially appear to have much in common, they really do have a lot in common. *Both* racial bigotry and obesity involve discrimination against racial minorities and women. *The Help* has a tag line that caught my eye. It's "Change begins with a whisper." This book is just a whisper.

But that's how change begins. As Dana Carpender said at the beginning of this chapter, *There is no short cut. It's a matter of reaching people one at a time, of telling our stories, of speaking out, of saying to the doctor, "Yes, I've lost weight and my blood work is better—it's because I'm on Atkins," of telling our friends, "I know, I ate a low fat diet, too, but it just made my diabetes worse; let me tell you what helped." It's like Gandhi said: you must be the change you want to see in the world.*

Here's a li'l old fat lady's dream…I go down to my local grocery store and wander among the aisles, marveling at the enormous bounty. There's the chip aisle with all the plastic bags trumpeting their superior nutritional value. The quantities of valuable proteins are listed along with the nutritional values for each of the nine essential amino acids. The wonderful fats they use to cook the chips in are the best in the world.

With *the New & Improved!* pioneering work of companies like Generation UCAN, the term "low-carb" is becoming outdated. Today, many high-carb foods no longer cause excessive insulin response like they did in the old days. Now, many of the processed food labels have the *lowPSS*SM logo. Products that have this logo are exempt from the Freedom Fund contribution, so I always keep an eye out for the *lowPSS*SM.

Next, I go over to the ice cream aisle. Instead of the two Safeway Select Watch'n Carbs flavors I treasured in the old days, there are now dozens and dozens of rich *New & Improved!* varieties. Do I want the Cheesecake Brownie or the Denali Chocolate Peanut Butter Moose Tracks or the Klondike Krunch? I just can't make up my mind. Then there are the new CarbSmart ice cream flavors, too. What a decision!

The baking and spice aisle now offers dozens of *New & Improved!* sweeteners, flours, and baking mixes. Oooh! There's my favorite triple chocolate brownie mix on sale! And I mustn't forget to pick up some *New & Improved!* Hamburger Helper.

Then I go to the bread and cereal aisles. The choice is almost as vast with the number of microbrewery–type, specialty, low PSS, high protein grain producers continuing to expand every day. The vegetable and fruit area is just as enticing with its expanse of low carbohydrate items. Each of the grocery store chains competes ferociously to offer the most unique nutritious varieties of low PSS fruits and vegetables. And, just like at Costco, I can sample many of the new items before I make my selection.

With the *New & Improved!* high protein grains and vegetables, the number of vegetarians and vegans has really increased. In the old days it was really difficult to get enough good quality protein with all the essential amino acids, but now that's all changed. Nowadays it's really easy to be vegetarian or vegan and still eat a delicious, low PSS diet that's also high in nutritious proteins and fats. Many of the grocery stores even have a complete "V" aisle.

The beverage aisle is next. Again, the number of *New & Improved!* soft drink options is enormous. Sadly, it's becoming harder to remember the days when Coke and Pepsi dominated the soda industry. Because they only focused on next quarter's earnings and didn't begin to offer *New & Improved!* soft drinks soon enough, they allowed other competitors like Zevia and Hansen's to gain valuable market share. So they're now at risk of joining other has-been names like Montgomery Ward, Oldsmobile, Mervyn's, Pontiac, F.W. Woolworth Company, Hummer, and Borders.

Then, I go to the meat section. With calories, fat, and cholesterol no longer being the villains, the meat section has exploded, along with the cheese selection. In the old days many of the supermarkets only stocked a few types of cheese. Now there's a whole separate cheese section with more than a hundred varieties. And for the gourmet cheese lover, there are the specialty cheese stores.

I almost forgot! I need to get pet food for Max, our 18-year-old dog and Bella, our 19-year-old cat. They are now becoming old, but they have had such wonderful, long, healthy lives. The *New & Improved!* pet foods are wonderful! The low PSS, high protein corn they now use contains many of the essential amino acids and essential fatty acids. What a difference that makes!

Let's see, tomorrow I have my Weight Watchers low PSS cooking class. Do I need to get anything to take to Weight Watchers? Yes! It's heavy whipping cream. And, before I forget, I need to make a note to place an online order with www.netrition.com and www.amazon.com for the gourmet low PSS specialty items that I can't get here.

I truly enjoy looking at my overflowing grocery cart that is filled with rich, delicious, low PSS foods that enable my family to be lean and healthy. Although my grocery bill has gone up, my discretionary income has actually increased because I no longer need to swallow so many of those little hard, tasteless prescription and over-the-counter medication pellets as I did in years past.

In the old days, after smoking was discovered to be harmful, a nationwide chain of 700-plus Smoker Friendly® stores sprung up. According to their website, "Smoker Friendly® is completely dedicated to the sale and promotion of cigarettes, cigars, all other tobacco products and related smoker's accessories in our stores through our friendly and knowledgeable store operators."[40] Then, when excessive sugars and carbohydrates turned out to be the *real* bad boys on the block, Sugar Friendly[SM] stores also began to pop up like mushrooms. So, whether your addiction is nicotine or PSS, there's a convenience store that's got what you're looking for. The majority of the Freedom Fund contributions now come from the Sugar Friendly[SM] stores.

Oops, I better finish up my grocery shopping, because I don't want to miss out on the VR (virtual reality) Alaskan bike ride that's showing at the family physical entertainment spa this evening. I'm not sure if my husband is touring Alaska with me or if he's playing quarterback for the Denver Broncos in the VR football game. The whole family just loves going to this particular physical entertainment spa because we've all made so many wonderful friends who share our same interests. The children have gotten really hooked on the VR bungee jumping and the VR zip line tours so I bet they'll resist going home when I'm ready to call it an evening.

Since it is so late, maybe the family should eat at McDonald's tonight. With their *New & Improved!* Happy Meals for the kids and their *New & Improved!* Value Meals for us adults, fast food no longer means junk food. I still can't believe the old McDonald's 22-ounce Chocolate McCafe Shake used to contain 147 grams of carbs![41] But, no more. McDonald's was the pioneer in *New & Improved!* fast food. Best of all, their *New & Improved!* french fries are absolutely wonderful. I'm starting to get hungry just thinking about them! Yes, we'll definitely go to McDonald's tonight. The kids will be thrilled. We'll go to the new location that opened last week—I just wish I had bought stock in McDonalds a few years ago.

It's a beautiful dream that I hope will someday become a reality.

This li'l old fat lady believes that America can change for the better. I believe we and our children can lead better lives. I believe that big business can improve next quarter's earnings. But we need to turn the kaleidoscope to see what *can* be rather than what *is*. We need to be able to raise ourselves above the ideas of the time. *We need to play America's game—Innovation.*

"The Americans were underdogs, but they were competitive. [Coach] Brooks suggested that a bronze medal was within reach."[42] Like the 1980 US Olympic hockey team's win over the Soviets, America needs to win the obesity game. Like the 1980 US Olympic hockey team's triumph over the Soviets, once we triumph over obesity, we can go on to capture the gold.

This book is just one more voice added to all the other low carb voices out there. I hope my Freedom Fund Marketing Strategies will complement the work of the low carb nutritional experts who are on the front lines. I hope this book will help other overweight and obese Americans regain their health and freedom. By changing the rules just a little, we can turn the tide of obesity. By changing our tune just a little, we can regain our freedom. As Martin Luther King said, "I have a dream." Let's play America's game—*Innovation*. Let's let freedom ring—again.

This book is dedicated to the victims of the September 11, 2001, World Trade Center disaster.

AUTHOR UPDATES

More key research has been published since this book was first written.

On page 121, there's a **Peggy Prediction**: Coloradoans are leaner than the rest of the country partly because they're higher. *Not drugs or alcohol high. Altitude high.* New scientific research validates this prediction and more:

> Recently, we've identified a strong association between obesity prevalence and altitude within the US . . . There was a **4-5 fold increase in obesity** prevalence at low altitude as compared with the highest altitude category after controlling for diet, activity level, smoking, demographics, temperature, and urbanization.[1]

> People living at higher altitudes have a lower chance of dying from ischemic heart disease and tend to live longer than others . . . Colorado, the highest state in the nation, is also the leanest state, the fittest state, and has the fewest deaths from heart disease and a lower incidence of colon and lung cancer compared to others.[2]

> If you look at people who live at high altitude around the world, incidents of most types of heart disease and stroke are much less.[3]

> Men and women who lived in counties at a higher altitude in the USA had a longer life expectancy.[4]

On page 132, there's a discussion regarding the economic development opportunities for rural communities that rank highly in natural amenities. But there was no research that specifically quantified the economic benefit. On March 11, 2015, the Center for Western Priorities published *THE GOLDEN RUSH: How Public Lands Draw Retirees and Create Economic Wealth.*[5] Here's the number. For every 100 retirees, 55 local jobs are created. Many smart rural communities are now rushing to attract seniors.

Pages 163-168 lay out the facts regarding a pasta product called Dreamfields that claims to have only *"5g Digestible Carbs Per Serving."* Here's the latest status.

> The makers of Dreamfields pasta have agreed to a $7.9 million class action lawsuit settlement over claims they falsely advertised the low-carb pasta as containing fewer digestible carbohydrates and as having a lower glycemic index than traditional pasta.[6]

References for Author Update:

1. Guest post from Jameson D. Voss, MD, by Travis Saunders, PhD, MSc, CEP, Obesity and Altitude, April 10, 2013. Research published in the International Journal of Obesity (2013) 37, 1407-1412.

2. University of Colorado School of Medicine, Public Release: 25-March-2011, http://www.eurekalert.org/pub_releases/2011-03/uocd-ssl032511.php.

3. Robert Roach, PhD, Altitude Research Center, University of Colorado School of Medicine. http://articles.chicagotribune.com/2011-09-07/health/sc-health-0907-living-at-altitude-20110907_1_heart-disease-high-altitude-lung-disease.

4. J Epidemiol Community Health (2011). doi:10.1136/jech. 2010.112938.

5. http://westernpriorities.org/goldenrush/.

6. http://topclassactions.com/lawsuit-settlements/closed-settlements/33102-dreamfields-pasta-class-action-settlement/.

LOW-CARB RESOURCES

BOOKS

Jeff S. Volek, PhD, RD, and Stephen D. Phinney, MD, PhD
- *The Art and Science of Low Carbohydrate Living* (2011)
- *The Art and Science of Low Carbohydrate Performance* (2012)
- *The New Atkins for a New You* (2010, along with author Eric C. Westman, MD, MHS)

Michael R. Eades, MD, and Mary Dan Eades, MD
- *Protein Power* (1999)
- *The Six-Week Cure for the Middle-Aged Middle* (2009)

Richard K. Bernstein, MD
- *The Diabetes Diet* (2005)
- *Dr. Bernstein's Diabetes Solution* (2011)

Gary Taubes
- Good Calories, Bad Calories (2008)
- Why We Get Fat (2011)

Jimmy Moore
- Livin' La Vida Low Carb (2005)
- 21 Life Lessons from Livin' La Vida Low Carb (2009)

Jeff O'Connell
- Sugar Nation (2011)

Jonny Bowden, PhD, CNS
- Living Low Carb (2010)

Dana Carpender
- 500 Low Carb Recipes (2002)
- How I Gave Up My Low-Fat Diet and Lost 40 Pounds (2003)
- 15-Minute Low-Carb Recipes (2003)
- The Low-Carb Barbecue Book (2004)
- 500 More Low-Carb Recipes (2004)
- 200 Low-Carb Slow Cooker Recipes (2005)
- Low-Carb Smoothies (2005)
- Dana Carpender's NEW Carb and Calorie Counter-Expanded, Revised, and Updated 4th Edition (2009)
- 1001 Low-Carb Recipes (2010)
- 300 15-Minute Low Carb Recipes (2011)
- 300 Low-Carb Slow Cooker Recipes (2011)
- 500 Paleo Recipes (Dec. 1, 2012)
- More

WEB SITES

- Nutrition & Metabolism Society — http://www.nmsociety.org
- CarbSmart — http://www.carbsmart.com
- Dana Carpender — http://holdthetoast.com
- Jimmy Moore — http://www.livinlavidalowcarb.com
- Andreas Eenfeldt, MD — http://www.dietdoctor.com
- Michael R. Eades, MD — http://www.proteinpower.com/drmike
- Jacqueline A. Eberstein, RN — http://www.controlcarb.com
- About.com — http://lowcarbdiets.about.com
- Obesity Action Coalition — http://www.obesityaction.org

NOTES

INTRODUCTION

1. *"…it rises from…bottom of rivers…"*: M.R. Eades, and M.D. Eades, *Protein Power* (New York: Bantam Books, 1999), pp. 3-4.

2. *"The yellow fever virus…seen in Africa."*: Wikipedia, accessed February 18,2012, http://en.wikipedia.org/wiki/Yellow_fever.

3. *"By 1977, when the notion…evolved independent of the science."*: G. Taubes, *Good Calories, Bad Calories* (New York: Anchor Books, 2008), p. 42.

4. *"[On] January 14, 1977,…from saturated fats."*: G. Taubes, *Good Calories, Bad Calories* (New York: Anchor Books, 2008), pp. 44-46.

5. *"Eat less saturated fat:…updated once every five years?"*: *Scientific American*, accessed July 12, 2012, http://www.scientificamerican.com/article.cfm?id=carbs-against-cardio.

6. *"The USDA Dietary Guidelines…and refined grains."*: USDA, accessed February 18, 2012, http://health.gov/dietaryguidelines/2010.asp.

CHAPTER 1: Just a Li'l Old Fat Lady Who Got Fed Up

1. *"In 2002, 230.6 million people… for over a year."*: BBC News, Published: 2003/02/19 08:37:34 GMT., accessed January 5, 2012, http://news.bbc.co.uk/2/hi/health/2779031.stm.

2. *The Federal Trade Commission…(eatright.org).*: FTC, accessed on July 12, 2012, http://www.ftc.gov/bcp/edu/microsites/whocares/weightloss.shtm.

3. *Let's take a recent Weight Watchers..."The Year to Believe."*: Weight Watchers, accessed on July 3, 2012, http://www.weightwatchers.com.

4. *That didn't stop U S News..."The best diet for losing weight is Weight Watchers."*: U S News, accessed on March 31, 2012, http://health.usnews.com/best-diet/best-weight-loss-diets/data.

5. *However, I did find... "...Congress should insist it do so."*: MedscapeWire article, accessed on January 15, 2012, http://www.medscape.com/viewarticle/411788.

6. *64% in 1999-2000*: National Center for Health Statistics, CDC, accessed on July 12, 2012, http://www.cdc.gov/nchs/products/pubs/pubd/hestats/obese/obse99.htm, accessed from epsl.asu.edu/ceru/Documents/NCHS_obesity.pdf.

7. *68.5% in 2007-2010*: http://www.cdc.gov/nchs/hus/contents2011.htm#074.

8. *Here's what CBS News has to say... "A review of 10...two years later."*: CBSnews.com, accessed on January 5, 2012, http://cbsnews.com/2102-204_162-664519.html?tag=contentMain;contentBody.

9. *The graph below...weight loss studies.*: J.W. Anderson and others, "Long-term weight-loss maintenance: a meta-analysis of US studies." *Am J Clin Nutr*, 2001; 74:579-84.

10. *At least for...$62 billion annually.*: New York Times, accessed on July 12, 2012, http://www.nytimes.com/2012/01/01/business/new-years-resolutions-recycled-are-a-boon-for-business.html.

11. *Figure 1*: J.W. Anderson and others, "Long-term weight-loss maintenance: a meta-analysis of US studies." *Am J Clin Nutr*, 2001;74:579-84.

12. *I should weigh 107-140 pounds.*: National Heart Lung and Blood Institute, U.S. Department of Health & Human Services, National Institutes of Health, accessed on July 12, 2012, 2012, http://www.nhlbi.nih.gov/guidelines/obesity/bmi_tbl.htm.

13. *a physiological condition...blood sugars.*: Wikipedia, accessed on June 22, 2012, http://en.wikipedia.org/wiki/Insulin_resistance.

14. *Creamy Chocolate shake.*: Slim-Fast, accessed on July 3, 2012, http://slim-fast.com/products/shakes/Lower-Carb-Vanilla-Cream.aspx.

15. *The first author...Gary Taubes.*: G. Taubes, *Good Calories, Bad Calories.* (New York: Anchor Books, 2008).

16. *The first author...Gary Taubes:* G. Taubes, *Why We Get Fat.* (New York: Kompf., 2011).

17. *first Dietary Goals for the United States.*: G. Taubes, *Good Calories, Bad Calories* (New York: Anchor Books, 2008), p. 44.

18. *This is not a diet book...maximize the benefits to our health.*": G. Taubes, *Why We Get Fat* (New York: Kompf, 2011), p. 201.

19. *A tragic 68.5%...overweight or obese.*: 68.5% in 2007-2010: http://www.cdc.gov/nchs/hus/contents2011.htm#074.

20. *Using 2010 Census data*: U S Census Bureau, accessed on July 1, 2012, http://2010.census.gov/2010census/data.

21. *"Today, about one in three...nearly triple the rate in 1963."*: American Heart Association, accessed on July 1, 2012, http://www.heart.org/HEARTORG/Getting-Healthy/Overweight-in-Children_UCM_304054_Article.jsp.

22. *70 million young Americans are overweight or obese.*: U S Census Bureau, accessed on July 1, 2012, http://2010.census.gov/2010census/data.

23. *totaled about $147 billion.*: Centers for Disease control, accessed on December 3, 2011, http://www.cdd.gov/obesity/causes/economics.html.

24. *medical costs per obese person of $2,741.*: Insurance Journal, accessed on July 12, 2012, http://insurancejournal.com/news/national/2012/04/10/242749.htm.

25. *average of about $3,600 per person.*: Medscape, accessed on January 26, 2012, http://www.medscape.com/viewarticle/751325.

26. *$861 to $957 billion by 2030*: V. L. Roger, and others, "2012 update: a report from the American Heart Association." *Circulation.* 2012: published online before print December 15, 2011, 10.1161/CIR.0b013e31823ac047.

27. *manufacturer named Specialized.*: Specialized, accessed on July 12, 2012, http://www.specialized.com.

28. *"Innovate or Die."*: ezinearticles.com, accessed on February 3, 2012, http://ezinearticles.com/?Specialized-Bikes---Innovate-Or-Die&id=5420486.

CHAPTER 2: Earth is *Not* at the Center of the Universe

1. *Galileo (1564-1642) was an Italian physicist*: Wikipedia, accessed on July 14, 2012, http://en.wikipedia.org/wiki/Galileo.

2. *"Calories measure energy...archaic in other contexts."*: The Office Diet, accessed on July 14, 2012, http://www.theofficediet.com/2008/06/09/understanding-calories-kilocalories-and-kilojoules.

3. *"In 1917,...sign of moral weakness."*: J. Bowden, *Living Low Carb* (New York: Sterling Publishing, 2010), p. 4.

4. *"The Krebs cycle...the body can obtain all its energy from protein and fats."*: Wikipedia, accessed on October 6, 2011, http://en.wikipedia.org/wiki/Citric_acid_cycle.

5. *OBESITY HALTING THE EPIDEMIC BY MAKING HEALTH EASIER.*: National Center for Chronic Disease Prevention and Health Promotion Division of Nutrition, Physical Activity, and Obesity, CDC, 4 page booklet, years 2009, 2010, and 2011.

6. *"A complete protein...corn protein, which is low in lysine and tryptophan."*: Wikipedia, accessed on April 27, 2012, and May 2, 2012, http://en.wikipedia.org/wiki/Complete_protein.

7. *"Essential fatty acids,...(a monounsaturated fatty acid)."*: Wikipedia, accessed on May 2, 2012, http://en.wikipedia.org/wiki/Essential_fatty-acid.

8. *...including The Diabetes Solution*: R. Bernstein, *The Diabetes Solution* (New York: Little, Brown and Company, 2011).

9. *...and The Diabetes Diet*: R. Bernstein, *The Diabetes Diet* (New York: Little, Brown and Company, 2005).

10. *"There are essential amino acids...but there is no such thing as an essential carbohydrate."*: R. Bernstein, *Dr. Bernstein's Diabetes Solution* (New York: Little, Brown and Company, 2011), p. 139.

11. *"Consume more of certain foods...and seafood"*: USDA, Accessed February 18, 2012, http://health.gov.dietaryguidelines/2010.asp.

12. *Including one called Living Low Carb*: J. Bowden, *Living Low Carb* (New York: Sterling Publishing, 2010).

13. *Inspirational books Livin' La Vida Low Carb*: J. Moore, *Livin' La Vida Low Carb* (2005).

14. *and 21 Life Lessons from Livin' La Vida Low-Carb.*: J. Moore, *21 Life Lessons from Livin' La Vida Low-Carb* (2009).

15. *...there's a new book*: J. Volek and S. Phinney, *The Art and Science of Low Carbohydrate Living* (2011).

16. *"I'm going to tell you about...best low-carb book I've ever read."*: M. Eades' blog, accessed March 14, 2012, http://www.proteinpower.com/drmike/saturated-fat/the-best-low-carb-book-in-print/#more-4765.

17. *"...I'm still going to gain weight."*: J. Bowden, *Living Low Carb* (New York: Sterling Publishing, 2010), p. 115.

18. *"...most Americans who are obese...low-carbohydrate diet."*: R. Bernstein, *Dr. Bernstein's Diabetes Solution* (New York: Little, Brown and Company, 2011), p. 141.

19. *"As for how much is too much protein,...higher in fat than protein."*: J. Volek and S. Phinney, *The Art and Science of Low Carbohydrate Living* (2011), p. 60.

20. *"This whole process...even type 2 diabetes."*: E. Westman, S. Phinney and J. Volek, *The New Atkins For a New You* (New York: Simon & Schuster, 2010), p. 22.

21. *"In the winter of 1928,...sunlight on our skin)."*: G. Taubes, *Good Calories, Bad Calories* (New York: Anchor Books, 2008), pp. 320-325.

CHAPTER 3: The *Real* Bad Boy on the Block

1. *most difficult time...never been a part of the mind-set.*: M.R. Eades and M.D. Eades, *Protein Power* (New York: Bantam Books, 1999), p. 326.

2. *"During my last visit,...emaciated arm covered with blotches to hold my hand."*: J. O'Connell, *Sugar Nation* (New York: Hyperion, 2011), p. 256.

3. *Here it is – read'm and weep.*: National Institute of Diabetes and Digestive and Kidney Diseases (NIDDK), National Diabetes Statistics, 2011, Accessed July 15, 2012, http://diabetes.niddk.nih.gov/dm/pubs/statistics/index.aspx.

4. *"Are we doomed…forestall further formation.":* M.R. Eades and M.D. Eades, *Protein Power* (New York: Bantam Books, 1999), p. 324.

5. *"Although it performs countless…dead in a matter of days or perhaps even hours.":* M.R. Eades and M.D. Eades, *Protein Power* (New York: Bantam Books, 1999), pp. 32-33.

6. *We love it. We go out of our way to find it…We were born this way.:* Robert H. Lustig, "Is Sugar Toxic?" CBS 60 Minutes, aired on April 1, 2012, http://www.cbsnews.com/video/watch/?id=7417238n&tag=mncol;lst;1.

7. *10% to 40% more…:* Wikipedia, accessed on July 15, 2012, http://en.wikipedia.org/wiki/Organic_food.

8. *world organic market growing by 20% a year.:* Wikipedia, accessed on July 15, 2012, http://en.wikipedia.org/wiki/Organic_food.

9. *Obesity rate in this country has gone from 12%…:* PubMed.gov, "Obesity in America. C. Menifield, *ABNF J.* 2008 Summer, 19(3):83-8.

10. *Obesity rate in this country….to 35.7%…:* C. Ogden and others, "Prevalence of Obesity in the United States, 2009-2010, U S Department of Health and Human Services, *NCHS Data Brief,* No. 82, January 2012.

11. *"A steady diet heavy in carbohydrates…and central obesity.":* M. R. Eades and M.D. Eades, *The Six-Week Cure for the Middle-Aged Middle* (New York: Three Rivers Press, 2009), p. 29.

12. *"Whether you eat…proportion to carbohydrate content.":* R. Bernstein, *Dr. Bernstein's Diabetes Solution* (New York: Little, Brown and Company, 2011), p. 140.

13. *"The Primary stimulator of insulin release…on insulin levels.":* J. Volek and S. Phinney, *The Art and Science of Low Carbohydrate Living* (2011), p. 78.

14. *Fat consumption produces…modest insulin response.:* J. Volek and S. Phinney, *The Art and Science of Low Carbohydrate Living* (2011), p. 210.

15. *"In this ecologic analysis,…pure starch carbohydrate with fewer nutrients.":* L. S. Gross and others. "Increased consumption of refined carbohydrates and the epidemic of type 2 diabetes in the United States: an ecological assessment," *Am J Clin Nutr* 2004; 79-774-9, accessed on February 16, 2012, http://www.ajcn.org.

16. Ibid.

17. Ibid.

18. *"Cupcakes may be addictive...a generation ago."*: R. Langreth and D. Stanford, "Fatty foods Addictive Like Cocaine in Growing Body of Scientific Research." *Bloomberg.com*, November 2, 2011, accessed on November 6, 2011, http://www.bloomberg.com/news/2011-11-02/fatty-foods-addictive-as-cocaine-in-growing-body-of-science.html.

19. *"...when dietary fat...add the fat."*: M. R. Eades and M.D. Eades, *Protein Power* (New York: Bantam, 1999), p. 39.

20. *"So what are carbohydrates?...after you digest it."*: R. Bernstein, *Dr. Bernstein's Diabetes Solution* (New York: Little, Brown and Company, 2011), pp. 139-140.

21. *Recently the corn growers...laugh or cry"*: Corn Refiners Association, www.corn.org, accessed on July 15, 2012, http://www.youtube.com/watch?v=I1SlBjbG7BQ.

22. *Jimmy refers to sugar as rat poison...*: J. Moore, *Livin' La Vida Low-Carb* (2005), p. 89.

23. *USDA Dietary Guidelines For Americans,2010*: USDA, accessed on July 15, 2012, http://www.cnpp.usda.gov/DGAs2010-PolicyDocument.htm.

24. *[USDA] document has increased in size to its current 112 pages.*: 1980 (11 pages), 1985 (13 pages), 1990 (14 pages), 1995 (25 pages), 2000 (44 pages), 2005 (84 pages), and 2010 (112 pages). Page counts are actual PDF document pages.

25. *U.S. Institute of Medicine...130 grams...*: Wikipedia, accessed on February 10, 2012, http://en.wikipedia.org/wiki/Low-carbohydrate_diet.

26. *The New Atkins...increasing that number.*: E. Westman, S. Phinney and J. Volek, *The New Atkins For A New You* (New York: Simon & Schuster, 2010), p. 15.

27. *"...the American Medical Association...potentially dangerous."*: Hearings Before the Select Committee on Nutrition and Human Needs of the United States Senate, Ninety-third Congress, First Session, Part 1 – Obesity and Fad Diets, Washington, D.C., April 12, 1973, Series 73/ND1, p. 2.

28. *A study of...recommends for weight loss."*: CNNMoney.com, "Low-carb dieters are way off target," accessed on January 24, 2012, http://money.cnn.com/2004/04/05/news/fortune500/food_carb/index.htm.

29. *"Bariatric surgery restricts…risks, including death."*: "Longitudinal Assessment of Bariatric Surgery (LABS)," National Institute of Diabetes and Digestive and Kidney Diseases (NIDDK), accessed October 17, 2011, http://win.niddk.nih.gov/publications.labs.htm.

30. *"Examples of side effects…(caused by lack of protein)."*: "Bariatric Surgery for Sever Obesity," National Institute of Diabetes and Digestive and Kidney Diseases (NIDDK), accessed October 17, 2011, http://win.niddk.nih.gov/publications/gastric.htm.

31. *"Currently, the most effective way…NIDDK established LABS."*: "Longitudinal Assessment of Bariatric Surgery (LABS)," National Institute of Diabetes and Digestive and Kidney Diseases (NIDDK), accessed October 17, 2011, http://win.niddk.nih.gov/publications.labs.htm.

32. *Shockingly, this surgery…significant regain."* : J. Odom and others, "Behavioral predictors of weight regain after bariatric surgery," *Obes Surg.* 2010 Mar; 20(3):349-56. Epub 2009 June 25. Accessed January 26, 2012, http://www.ncbi, nlm.nih.gov/pubmed/19554382.

33. *"New research…contributed grant support."*: M. Marchione, *The Associated Press,* Monday, March 26, 2012, 11:44 AM EDT, accessed March 27, 2012, http://www.mycenturylink.com/news/read.php?id=2341041&ps=1018&cat=&cps=0&lang=en.

34. *The Introduction chapter…very good answer for everyone else.)"*: R. Bernstein, *The Diabetes Diet* (New York: Little, Brown and Company, 2005).

35. *"In conclusion…adolescents with morbid obesity in the future."*: R. Weiss, "Bariatric Surgery in Adolescents—The Sooner the Better?" Nature Publishing Group, posted : 06/21/2010, accessed January 15, 2012, http://www.medscape.com/viewarticle/723126.

36. *And Magdalena Plecka Östlund, MD increased alcohol concentrations."*: C. Helwick, MedScape Medical News, Digestive Disease Week (DDW) 2011: Abstract 266, Presented May 7, 2011, accessed on January 26, 2012, http://www.medscape.com/viewarticle/742434.

37. *By 6 years, …terms of fractures."*: C. Frincu-Mallos, MedScape Medical News, ENDO 2009: The Endocrine Society Annual Meeting: Abstract OR07-4. Presented June 10, 2009, http://www.medscape.com/viewarticle/704264.

38. *"Women under age 65…[from surgery]."*: "Bone mineral density test," PubMed Health, accessed on February 2, 2012, http://www.ncbi.nlm.hih.gov/pubmed-health/MPH0004464.

39. *Ibid.*

40. *My T score was +1.6.*: Study: Bone Densitometry. July 2, 2008. Indication: Post-menopausal. AP Spine (L1-L4)-T-Score of 3.0, Total Hip (L)-T-Score of 1.6. "Under the guidelines of the International Society for Clinical Densitometry, the lowest T-score of the spine or hip…is used to determine the classification."

41. *…average cost for bariatric surgery is $20,000-$25,000.*: "Bariatric Surgery for Severe Obesity," National Institute of Diabetes and Digestive and Kidney Diseases (NIDDK), accessed October 17, 2011, http://win.niddk.nih.gov/publications/gastric.htm.

42. *…the price tag can go as high as $69,960.*: "Complications and Costs for Obesity Surgery Declining," Agency for Healthcare Research and Quality, US Department of Health and Human Services, Press Release Date: April 29, 2009, accessed on April 23, 2012, http:www/ahrq.gov/news/press/pr2009/barsurgpr.htm.

43. *…family coverage is $15,520 (200+ workers).*: "Employer Health Benefits 2011 Annual Survey," September 2011, The Kaiser Family Foundation and Health Research & Educational Trust, Publication #8225, p. 23, at www.kff.org.

44. *…estimate for bariatric surgeries in2008 was 220,000.*: "Longitudinal Assessment of Bariatric Surgery (LABS)," National Institute of Diabetes and Digestive and Kidney Diseases (NIDDK), accessed October 17, 2011, http://win.niddk.nih.gov/publications.labs.htm.

45. *"The 6-month post-surgical death rate… was 0.5%."*: "Complications and Costs for Obesity Surgery Declining," Agency for Healthcare Research and Quality, US Department of Health and Human Services, Press Release Date: April 29, 2009, accessed on April 23, 2012, http:www/ahrq.gov/news/press/pr2009/barsurgpr.htm.

46. *…the NIDDK is now quoting a 0.3% death rate.*: "NIH Study Finds Low Short-term Risks After Bariatric Surgery for Extreme Obesity," NIH News, US Department of Health and Human Services, Released July 30, 2009, accessed on April 25, 2012, http://www.hig.gov.news/health/jul2009/niddk-30.htm.

47. *'the incidence of bariatric deaths in New York City is practically unknowable for us.'*: J. Goldstein, "State probes weight-loss deaths at NYU. New York Post, June 13,

2010, 5:54 AM, accessed on April 25, 2012, http://www.nypost.com/p/news/local/horror_stories_follow_lap_band_surgery_JPHaUeuhbIANvH6orXEfeP.

48. *"Bariatric procedures …often around $4,000.":* Ibid.

49. *"Bariatric surgeries have exploded in popularity.":* Ibid.

CHAPTER 4: My Deal With The Devil

1. *(This is a term…happen suddenly and unexpectedly.):* M. Gladwell, *The Tipping Point* (New York: Little, Brown and Company, 2002).

2. *They finally gave up and…offers the product.:* Phone call to Land-O-Lakes on 800-878-9762, 7/3/12, 12:05pm, UPC 3450063165.

3. *So, a cup of Splenda actually contains 24g of carbs.:* About.com, accessed on May 2, 2012, http://lowcarbdiets.about.com/od/products/a/liquidsplenda.htm.

4. *"Since the manufacturer of Splenda has held back…sucralose in liquid forms.":* About.com, accessed on May 2, 2012, http://lowcarbdiets.about.com/od/products/a/liquidsplenda.htm.

5. *Unfortunately, when I looked…ingredients listed.:* Manufacturer's web site. Accessed on July 11, 2012, http://www.intheraw.com/products/stevia-in-the-raw.

6. *There's no sugar in sheep's clothing listed…nutrition label.:* Truvia.com, accessed on July 3, 2012, http://truvia.com/about/ingredients/.

7. *Lead pollution from engine exhaust…particularly harmful effects on children.:* Wikipedia, accessed on July 17, 2012, http://en.wikipedia.org/wiki/Leaded_gasoline.

8. *"GM started marketing its Ethyl"…still being used in the developing world.":* B. Kovarik, "Ethyl War Forbidden Fuel and Public Poison," accessed on January 6, 2012, http://www.radford.edu/~wkovarik/ethylwar/overview.html.

9. *…coverage to be $15,520 (200+ workers).:* "Employer Health Benefits 2011 Annual Survey," September 2011, The Kaiser Family Foundation and Health Research & Educational Trust, Publication #8225, p. 23, at www.kff.org.

10. *But they've added so much sugar…Honey Nut Cheerios!*: Walmart.com, accessed on July 3, 2012, http://www.walmart.com/ip/Honey-Nut-Cheerios-Cereal-17-oz/10311277.

11. *A single 25 biscuit serving…41 grams of carbs.*: Walmart.com, accessed on July 3, 2012, http://www.walmart.com/ip/Kellogg-s-Frosted-Mini-Wheats-Bite-Size-Strawberry-Delight-Cereal-21-oz/19757536.

12. *…"Sugar Free" ice cream topping had 11g of carbs.*: Smucker's. Accessed on July 3, 2012, http://www.smuckers.com/products/ProductDetail.aspx?groupId=4&categoryId=50&flavorId=751.

13. *…Smuckers Carmel ice cream topping contains 30g of carbs.*: Smucker's. Accessed on July 3, 2012, http://www.smuckers.com/products/ProductDetail.aspx?groupId=4&categoryId=48&flavorId=117.

14. *…there's a company…product called Carbquik.*: Carbalose.com, accessed on July 17, 2012, http://www.tovaindustries.com/carbalose/carbquik-faq.html.

15. *"…we stand by our packaging labels on both the Carbalose Flour and Carbquik. The nutritional information, including carb counts are correct.":* E-mail from Tova Industries representing that the owner had confirmed this information, August 17, 2011, 3:13 pm MST.

16. *Carbquik (96g) has 48g of carbs of which 42g are fiber.*: Netrition. Accessed on July 3, 2012, http://www.netrition.com/tova_carbquik_page.html#NUTFACTS.

17. *A cup of Bisquick (120g) has a carb count of 78g of which 3g are fiber.*: Walmart. Accessed on July 3, 2012, http://www.walmart.com/ip/Bisquick-Pancake-Mix-96-oz/10311530.

18. *…diabetic's blood sugars significantly when consumed by the tablespoon.*: R. Bernstein. *Dr. Bernstein's Diabetes Solution.* 2011 (New York: Little, Brown and Company, 2011), p. 150.

19. *…states xylitol will not raise your insulin level.*: J. Volek and S. Phinney. *The Art and Science of Low Carbohydrate Living* (2011), p. 225.

20. *Approved by FDA in October 2003. Dr. Bernstein unsure of PSS impact.*: R. Bernstein. *Dr. Bernstein's Diabetes Solution.* 2011 (New York: Little, Brown and Company, 2011), p. 150.

21. *And Cargill is testing out Treha (trehalose) that might be "incorporated as part of a sports beverage system.":* Cargill Foods. Accessed on July 17, 2012, http://www.cargill-foods.com/na/en/products/sweeteners/specialty-sweeteners/treha.trehalose/index.jsp.

CHAPTER 5: Exercise Should Be a Four-Letter Word

1. *"There are no data on weight loss when you go to a health club either.":* T. Wadden. "Diet Plan Success Tough To Weigh." CBSnews.com, access on January 5, 2012, http://cbsnews.com/2102-204_162-664519.html?tag=contentMain;contentBody.

2. *…only about 31%…at least 5 days per week.":* NIH. WIN – Statistics. Accessed on January 5, 2012, http://win.niddk.nig.gov.statistics/index.htm#causes.

3. *In 2012, Leadville was nationally rated second…:* True West Magazine. Accessed on July 17, 2012, http://www.truewestmagazine.com/jcontent/living-the-dream/living-the-dream/true-western-towns/4462-2012-top-ten-true-western-towns.

4. *… Over The Hill Gang for 50+ year old skiers.:* Copper Mountain. Accessed on July 17, 2012, http://www.coppercolorado.com/winter/ski_and_ride_school/on_the_hill_gang.

5. *"Although exercise…fitness leads to further fitness.":* R. Bernstein. *Dr. Bernstein's Diabetes Solution* (New York: Little, Brown and Company, 2011), p. 225.

6. *"Why write this booklet now?...power-to-weight ratios.":* J. Volek and S. Phinney. *The Art and Science of Low Carbohydrate Performance* (2012), pp. 4-5.

7. *"Regular exercise…magic elixir of youth.":* M. R. Eades and M.D. Eades. *Protein Power* (New York: Bantam Books, 1999), p. 203.

8. *…14 different yoga…Viniyoga, and Yin.":* Women's Health Magazine. Accessed on February 3, 2012, http://www.womenshealthmag.com/yoga/types-of-yoga.

9. *"The style is best-known…Goldie Hawn).":* Women's Health Magazine. Accessed on February 3, 2012, http://www.womenshealthmag.com/yoga/bikram-yoga.

10. *"Despite the proven health benefits…aerobic exercise training.":* N. P. Greene and others. American College of Sports Medicine. Medicine and Science in Sports and Exercise. 2009;41(9):1808-1815. Accessed on January 14, 2012, http://www.med-scape.com/viewarticle/708917.

11. *Colorado has 54 mountain peaks that are higher than 14,000'.*: 14ers.com, accessed on July 17, 2012, http://www.14ers.com.

CHAPTER 6: Your Best Friends Can Be Your Worst Enemies

1. *"Don't let the noise of others' opinion drown…follow your heart and tuition."*: C. Duhigg, "With time running short, Jobs managed his farewells." The New York Times, October 6, 2011, accessed on October 10, 2011, http://www.msnbc, msn/id/44815146.

2. *Overeaters Anonymous' web site states…in over 75 countries.*: Overeaters Anonymous, accessed July 17, 2012, http://www.oa.org/newcomers/about-oa.

3. *"Weight-loss surgery is a…severe obesity."*: Obesity Action Coalition, accessed on April 26, 2012, http://www.obesityaction.org/obesity/-treatments/bariatric-surgery.

4. *"Ethyl alcohol,…body does not convert it into glucose."*: R. Bernstein. *Dr. Bernstein's Diabetes Solution* (New York: Little, Brown and Company, 2011), p. 142.

5. *…and Michael. R. Eades…weight is normal.*: M. R. Eades and M.D. Eades, *The Six-Week Cure for the Middle-Aged Middle* (New York: Three Rivers Press, 2009), p. 149.

CHAPTER 7: Where You Live Can Make a Difference

3. *A 1999 United States…natural amenities.*: Natural Amenities Scale, USDA, accessed on July 17, 2012, http://www.ers.usda.gov/data-products/natural-amenities-scale.aspx.

4. *The Centers for Disease Control…rates at the county level.*: CDC, http://apps.nccd.cdc.gov/DDT_STRS2/CountyPrevalenceData.aspx?mode=OBS.

5. *…totaled about $147 billion.*: Centers for Disease control, accessed on December 3, 2011, http://www.cdd.gov/obesity/causes/economics.html.

6. *…$861 to $957 billion by 2030.*: V. L. Roger, and others, "2012 update: a report from the American Heart Association." *Circulation.* 2012: published online before print December 15, 2011, 10.1161/CIR.0b013e31823ac047.

7. *According to the CDC, the obesity…32.4% for whites.*: K. M. Flegal, and others. *JAMA* 2010; 303:235-241.

8. *"This study shows that obese subjects lose weight at high altitudes.":* F. J. Lippl and others. *Obesity* (2010) 18, 675-681,dol:10,1038/0by.2009.509.

9. *"Mechanisms of Obesity-induced Male Infertility...air-cooling devices during sleep.":* K. P. Phillips and N. *Tanphaichitr, Expert Rev Endocrinol Metab.* 2010:5(2):229-251, accessed on January 26, 2012, http://www.medscape.com/viewarticle/719489.

10. *"Exenatide: From the Gila Monster to the Pharmacy...reduction of food intake.":* C. Triplitt and E. Chiquette. *J Am Pharm Assoc.* 2006:46(1):44-55. American Pharmacists Association, accessed on January 26, 2012, http://www.medscape.com/viewarticle/521830.

11. *Colorado has the highest mean elevation (6,800') of any state...Mississippi's mean altitude is 300'.:* Wikipedia, accessed on November 28, 2011, http://en.wikipedia.org/wiki/List_of_U.S._states_by_elevation.

12. *In 1990, the Colorado obesity rate was 6.9%.:* United Health Foundation. America's Health Rankings, accessed on July 18, 2012, http://www.americashealthrankings.org./CO/Obesity/1990.

13. *...but in 2010 it was 21%.:* CDC, 2010 State Obesity Rates, accessed on July 18, 2012, http://www.cdc.gov/obesity/data/adult.html.

14. *If current trends continue, by 2020, 29% of Coloradans will be obese.:* Colorado Department of Health and Environment, Colorado Physical Activity and Nutrition State Plan 2010.

15. *"Overall, the proportion of...companies using penalties is expected to climb... National Workrights Institute.":* J. Mincer, "Firms to Charge Smokers, Obese More for Healthcare, Rueters Health Information, accessed on January 15, 2012, http://www.medscape.com/viewarticle/752653.

16. *"But the best news might be for older males...to every 100 women in that age group.":* S. Holland, "2010 Census shows more elderly than ever before in the U.S., CNN, 2011-11-30T18:04:50Z, accessed on December 1, 2011, http://222.cnn.com/2011/11/30/us/census-elderly/index.html.

17. *"Smoking, Obesity Slash American Life...men, it was 84 counties.":* E. Landau, "Smoking, Obesity Slash American Life Expectancy," CNN, 7:07 am PDT June 16, 2011, accessed on December 3, 2011, http:www.10news.com/print/28249428/detail.html.

18. *...40 years...are killing off the older obese women more quickly than the older obese men.*: K. M. Flegal, and others. *JAMA* 2010;303:235-241.

19. *"Falling behind: life expectancy in US counties from 2000 to 2007 in an international context."*: S. Kulkarni and others. *Population Health Metrics* 2011,9:16.

20. *March 2011 report from Harvard...under age 25 suffered only a 20.6% decline in mobility.*: G. Yedinak, "Seniors are Staying in Homes Longer, Less Like to Sell," accessed on December 3, 2011, http://seniorhousingnews.com/2011/05/16/seniors-are-staying-in-homes-longer-less-likely-to-sell.

21. *"Medicare costs to reduce Social Security increase..."*: S. Ohlemacher, Associated Press, October 19, 2011 6:12 PM EDT.

22. *"Medicare back on the brink over cuts to doctors."*: R. Alonso-Zaldivar, Associated Press, November 28, 2011 3:37 AM EST.

23. *"Despite competition and choice...comparable private insurance premiums."*: J. McCarter, Daily Kos, Monday, January 9, 2012 1:20 PM EST.

24. *"The SGR is the annual growth rate...Job Creation Act of 2012."*: B. Herman, Becker Hospital Review, May 9, 2012.

25. *On May 9, 2012, U S Representatives Allyson Schwartz and Joe Heck released the Medicare Physician Payment Innovation Act of 2012 – a bill...military operations in Iraq and Afghanistan.*: B. Herman, Becker Hospital Review, May 9, 2012.

26. *Medical Group Management Association (MGMA) research indicates that...patients.*: M. Vuletich, MGMA blog, November 16, 2010.

27. *"Mayo [Clinic]...will no longer accept Medicare patients...dropping out of the program."*: The Wall Street Journal, WSJ.com Review & Outlook, January 8, 2010.

28. *... whereas 95-100% is considered normal.*: Mayo Clinic. Original Article: http://www.mayoclinic.com/hypoxemia/MY00219.

29. *The Denver Colorado metropolitan area has a population of almost 2.5 million...*: (includes Denver county with 600,158, Jefferson county with 534,543, Arapahoe county with 572,003, Adams county with 441,603, Douglas county with 285,465, and Broomfield county with 55,889). 2010 Census, accessed on Aug. 7, 2012, http://quickfacts.census.gov/qfd/states/08/08005.html.

30. *...an analysis of cost data from several major national databases confirms...BMI between 25 and 27.*: Medscape, accessed on January 26, 2012, http://www.medscape.com/viewarticle/751325.

31. *The NIH confirms the same thing for diabetes - the health care costs are over twice as high for a diabetic.*: National Institute of Diabetes and Digestive and Kidney Diseases (NIDDK), National Diabetes Statistics, 2011, Accessed July 15, 2012, http://diabetes.niddk.nih.gov/dm/pubs/statistics/index.aspx.

32. *In a study titled, "The Benefits ...with little or no additional lifetime medical spending.":* D. Goldman and others, "The Benefits of Risk Factor Prevention in Americans Aged 51 Years and Older, American Journal of Public Health. 2009;99(1):2096, Posted 01/25/2010, accessed on January 15, 2012, http://www.medscape.com/viewarticle/71437.

33. *The Colorado Department of Public Health has a list of more than 100 facilities and I'm not sure that's all of them.*: Colorado Assisted Living Facilities which operate a secured environment specializing in services for residents with dementia and memory loss, http://www.cdphe.state.co.us/hf/alr/securebedsalr.pdf.

34. *"As it turns out, both Alzheimer's disease and most cancers... increase the risk of Alzheimer's disease.":* G. Taubes, *Why We Get Fat* (New York: Kompf, 2011), p. 198.

35. *...Associated Press report states, "US wants effective Alzheimer's treatment by 2025.":* The AP reports...$1 trillion in medical and nursing home expenditures.: L. Neergaard, Associated Press, January 17, 2012: 2:04 AM EST.

36. *"We found that overweight men were three times more likely to...have their cancer spread.":* K. Doheny, American Urological Association annual meeting, May 14-19, 2011, Washing D.C., accessed on January 26, 2012, http://medscape.com/viewarticle/742932.

37. *"Obesity greatly increased the risk for metastasis, as well as for recurrence and death...an almost double risk for cancer recurrence and death, compared with all the other patients.":* Z. Chustecka, Arch Surg. 2009;144;216-221. Abstract, accessed on January 26, 2012, http://www.medscape.com/viewarticle/589812.

38. *...the CDC now reports that 50 million U S adults... "Obesity is associated with incident knee...arthritis.":* Y. J. Cheng and others, Centers for Disease Control and Prevention, accessed on January 5, 2012, http://www.cdc.gov/Features/dsArthritisObesity.

39. *"Senior citizens have become the largest and fastest-growing segment of the U.S. population... influences everything from consumer behavior to health-care costs...":* The Wall Street Journal, WSJ.com, November 30, 2011, 4:04 PM ET.

40. *"Natural Amenities Drive Rural Population Change" that states, "Average 1970-96 population...the top quarter of the amenities index.":* D. McGranahan, USDA Economic Research Service, accessed July 17, 2012, http://ers.usda.gov/publications/aer-agricultural-economic-report/aer781.aspx.

41. *Median nonmetropolitan county change, 1970-2010, by level of natural amenities:* USDA Economic Research Service, accessed on July 19, 2012, http://www.ers.usda.gov/topics/rural-economy-population/natural-amenities/measures-of-natural-amenities-and-their-research-use.aspx.

CHAPTER 8: Pearls of Wisdom

1. *In June 2011, the USDA replaced MyPyramid....as the government's primary food group symbol.:* National Agricultural Library, USDA, accessed on August 5, 2012. http://fnic.nal.usda.gov/dietary-guidance/myplatefood-pyramid-resources/usda-myplate-food-pyramid-resources.

2. *Jonny Bowden's Healthy Low-Carb Live Pyramid:* J. Bowden. *Living Low Carb* (New York: Sterling Publishing Co. Inc., 2010), p. 379.

3. *...let's take a look....Duke University Medical Center:* E. Westman. Lifestyle Medicine Clinic at Duke University Medical Center. Nutrition & Metabolism Society Symposium, April 21-22, 2012.

4. *...Gary Taubes also advocates the Duke University dietary strategy:* G. Taubes, *Why We Get Fat* (New York: Alfred A. Knopf, 2011), pp. 219-225.

5. *"They said they read this little book, the Atkins Book...And Yet what I had heard was that it couldn't work and it was unhealthy.":* S. Schlender. Interview with Dr. Eric Westman, March 24, 2010. Accessed on July 26, 2012, http://www.meandmydiabetes.com/2010/03/24/eric-westman-duke-university-md-on-low-carb-high-fat-new-atkins-diet-password-protected-until-march-24th.

6. *Lifestyle Medicine Clinic Duke University Medical Center "No Sugar, No Starch" Diet:* Getting Started: E. Westman. Lifestyle Medicine Clinic at Duke University Medical Center. Nutrition & Metabolism Society Symposium, April 21-22, 2012.

7. *…let's take a look at a couple of pictures from The Art and Science of Low Carbo-hydrate Living*: J. Volek and S. Phinney. *The Art and Science of Low Carbohydrate Living* (2011), p. 208.

8. *"Honor the 'Schwatka Imperative'…the positive changes in one's life become positive-ly reinforcing."*: J. Volek and S. Phinney. *The Art and Science of Low Carbohydrate Living* (2011), pp. 237-245.

CHAPTER 9: Foods and Recipes That Will Knock Your Socks and 90 Pounds Off

1. *"…when dietary fat…add the fat."*: M. R. Eades and M.D. Eades, *Protein Power* (New York: Bantam, 1999), p. 39.

2. *The phrase snake oil is…"snake oil salesmen" became a tag for charlatans*: Wikipedia, Accessed on August 7, 2012, http://en.wikipedia.org/wiki/Snake_oil_salesman.

3. *"With only 5 grams of digestible carbs,…Dreamfields offers many health benefits and has been clinically tested to establish digestible carbohydrate levels."*: Box of Dream-fields Pasta Elbows, Apr172013 X1 J 04.

4. *"A scandalous controversy of sorts… only way YOU can know how the Dreamfields pasta is going to impact you is to simply do the test for yourself…"*: Jimmy Moore Blog, accessed on July 27, 2012, http://livinlavidalowcarb.com/blog/dreamfields-presi-dent-mike-crowley-we-stand-behind-the-nutritional-claims-of-our-product/10785.

5. *Withdrawn*: Screenprint of American Diabetes Care study of Dreamfields Pasta, accessed on July 27, 2012, http://care.diabetesjournals.org/content/34/9/2138.full.

6. *How I Gave Up My Low-Fat Diet and Lost 40 Pounds "*: D. Carpender, *How I Gave Up My Low-Fat Diet and Lost 40 Pounds*, (Massachusetts, Fair Winds Press, 2003).

7. *Since sweetness is one of the five basic senses and is almost universally regarded as a pleasurable experience…*: Wikipedia, accessed on July 27, 2012, http://en.wikipedia.org/wiki/Sweetness.

8. *Here's an example of pure frustration. Hershey's owns Mauna Loa which makes dark chocolate sugar free covered Mauna Loa macadamia nuts…Can I order them from Amazon.com? Nope.*: Phone call made to Hershey's at (800) 468-1714 on August 9, 2012. UPC is 7299205580, 4 oz. bag.

9. *According to their web site, LorAnn Oils is a family owned and operated business...and they currently offer oils for foods, aromatherapy and spa, and fragrances.*: LorAnn Oils, Inc., accessed on July 28, 2012, http://www.lorannoils.com/c-74-our-company.aspx.

10. *The only ding I must give Diversified Distributing is...*: Diversified Distributing. Accessed on August 8, 2012, http://www.yourfoodstore.com/spices.php. E-mail sent on August 8, 2012.

11. *So, I plucked out a smoothie called a Power Up! Protein Shake... and doctored it up a bit.*: M. R. Eades and M.D. Eades, *The Six-Week Cure for the Middle-Aged Middle* (New York: Three Rivers Press, 2009), pp. 115-117.

12. *Here's a sauce recipe that is inspired by one of Dana's cookbooks.*: D. Carpender, 500 Low-Carb Recipes (Massachusetts: Fair Winds Press, 2002), p. 240.

13. *I took a recipe from Michael R. Eades, MD and Mary Dan Eades, MD's book... and doctored it up a bit.*: M. R. Eades and M.D. Eades, *The Six-Week Cure for the Middle-Aged Middle* (New York: Three Rivers Press, 2009), p. 257.

CHAPTER 10: Just One Fourth of a Penny

1. *"The first sign of an upset in the making came in at the end of the first period... taking advantage of tired Soviet legs.":* J. Fitzpatrick, Miracle on Ice: American Hockey's Defining Moment, About.com, accessed on June 26, 2012, http://proice-hockey.about.com/cs/history/a/miracle_on_ice_2.htm.

2. *The Americans were underdogs, but they were competitive.*: J. Fitzpatrick, Miracle on Ice: American Hockey's Defining Moment, About.com, accessed on June 26, 2012, http://proicehockey.about.com/cs/history/a/miracle_on_ice.htm.

3. *"Play your game. Play your game. Play your game. Play your game.":* J. Lapointe, BackTalk; Remembering Herb Brooks: A Moment in Time, The New York Times, accessed on June 26, 2012, http://www.nytimes.com/2003/08/17/sports.

4. *...E. Jerome McCarthy, proposed a four Ps...throughout the world.*: Wikipedia, accessed on June 4, 2012, http://en.widipedia.org/wiki/Marketing_mix.

5. *...completely alter the marketing mix...*: Wikipedia, accessed on June 4, 2012, http://en.widipedia.org/wiki/Marketing_mix.

6. *In a study, Point-of-purchase Price and Education Intervention…education campaign phase.*: J. Block, and others. Point-of-purchase Price and Education Intervention to Reduce Consumption of Sugary Soft Drinks, American Journal of Public Health, 2010;100(8):1427-1433, accessed on January 15, 2012, http://www.medscape.com/viewarticle/736444.

7. *Malcolm Gladwell's book, The Tipping Point*: M. Gladwell, *The Tipping Point* (New York: Little, Brown and Company, 2002).

8. *…one gallon of gasoline has a nationwide average of almost 49¢hidden…has $3.46 hidden in the price.*: The Tax Foundation, accessed on September 1, 2011, http://www.taxfoundation.org.

9. *Americans bought nearly $1.5 billion worth of lotto tickets for a single $640 Mega Millions jackpot.*: M. Beck, Associated Press, March 30, 2012 4:34 PM EDT.

10. *It's a fund to help offset the $300 billion…*: B. Herman, Becker Hospital Review, May 9, 2012.

11. *"Medicare back on the brink over cuts to doctors."*: R. Alonso-Zaldivar, Associated Press, November 28, 2011 3:37 AM EST.

12. *"Medicare costs to reduce Social Security increase."*: S. Ohlemacher, Associated Press, October 19, 2011 6:12 PM EDT.

13. *With an estimated 311,591,917…*: Population 2011 estimate, U.S. Census Bureau, QuickFacts.

14. *(51% of the $911 billion Health and Human Services 2011 Budget).*: U S Department of Health and Human Services, p. 1, accessed on July 21, 2012, http://www.hhs.gov/about/budget/fy2011/#Brief.

15. *"An increased consumption of refined carbohydrates and the epidemic of type 2 diabetes in the United States: an ecologic assessment,"*: L. S. Gross and others. "Increased consumption of refined carbohydrates and the epidemic of type 2 diabetes in the United States: an ecological assessment," *Am J Clin Nutr* 2004; 79-774-9, accessed on February 16, 2012, http://www.ajcn.org.

16. Ibid.

17. *"Obesity is an extremely common problem… risk of diabetes, liver problems and joint pain."*: ASPCA we are their voice, accessed on March 22, 2012, http://www.aspc.org.

18. *"A recent survey indicates over 50% of America's pet population is overweight or obese…and Gourmet Dog.*: PetMD, The Overweight Pet, accessed on March 22, 2012, http://www.pedmd.com/dog/nutrition/evr_dg_identify_overweight_pet.

19. *The Humane Society approximates that Americans own 78.2 million dogs and 86.4 million cats, or 164.6 million dogs and cats.*: The Humane Society of the United States, accessed on March 22, 2012, http://www.humanesociety.org.

20. *The ASPCA even talks about, "Owner Behavior Modification.".*: ASPCA we are their voice, accessed on March 22, 2012, http://www.aspc.org.

21. *Dr. Vernon has participated in the training of 10 nationally ranked agility dogs including the #2 beagle (2 years) and #1 Norfolk Terrier (8 years)…*: Innovative Metabolic Solutions, Scribd, accessed on July 3, 2012, https://www.myimsonline.com/news/Presentation-by-Dr-Mary-Vernon-at-KU-Medical-Center.

22. *"My dogs eat the highest protein dog food that's available.".*: Innovative Metabolic Solutions, lecture on YouTube, accessed on July 3, 2012, https://www.myimsonline.com/news/Presentation-by-Dr-Mary-Vernon-at-KU-Medical-Center.

23. *A McDonalds Big Mac has 45g of PSS (carbs).*: McDonald's USA NutritionFacts for Popular Menu Items, PDF, saved on March 30, 2012.

24. *…3g of PSS (carbs) but 10 grams of essential proteins contained in a Church's fried chicken leg.*: Church's Chicken Nutrition & Allergen Information, PDF, saved on April 1, 2012.

25. *…Mary Dan Eades, MD, say in their book,…Middle.*: M.R. Eades and M.D. Eades. *The Six-Week Cure for the Middle-Aged Middle* (New York: Three Rivers Press, 2009), p. 70.

26. *"The worst hamburger we have is better …in my opinion.".*: Innovative Metabolic Solutions, lecture on YouTube, accessed on July 3, 2012, https://www.myimsonline.com/news/Presentation-by-Dr-Mary-Vernon-at-KU-Medical-Center.

27. *"Daniel Gallie, professor of biochemistry at UC Riverside in the United States, has successfully doubled the protein and oil content of corn grain, a discovery…and who normally avoid corn in their diets.".*: T. Young and others, Senescence-induced expression of cytokinin reverses pistil abortion during maize flower development, The Plant Journal (2004) 38, 910-922, Food Navigator-USA.com, 26-Sep-2005, accessed on February 25, 2012, http://www.foodnavigator-usa.com/content/vew/print/87591.

28. *"Conventional rice has barely 7-8 percent protein, while the high-protein rice (HPR) contains as much as 14-15 percent protein…also uses 60% less water to grow.":* DNA/Shilpa C B / Tuesday, November 15, 2011 12:28 IST, accessed on February 25, 2012, http://www.dnaindia.com.

29. *"Scientists at the National Institute for Plant Genome Research in New Delhi (India) are planning to seek regulatory approval…nutritionally rich protein.":* S. Chakraborty and others. "Next-generation protein-rich potato expressing the seed protein gene AmA1 is a result of proteome rebalancing in transgenic tuber," PNAS October 12, 2010, vol. 107, no. 41, 17533-17538, K. S. Jayaraman, Nature India Science News, doi:10.1038/nindia.2010.127; Published online 21 September 2010.

30. *In 2006, the United States alone grew 53% of the global transgenic crops.:* U S Department of Energy Office of Science, Office of Biological and Environmental Research, Human Genome Program, accessed on August 6, 2012, http://www.ornl.gov/sci/techresources/Human_Genome/elsi/gmfood.shtml.

31. *"Dr. Chad Hutchinson, from Florida University, and HZPC, a Dutch seed company, have been working on developing a new carb-friendly potato…flavor is exceptional.":* Medical News Today, May 30, 2004, accessed on February 18, 2012, http://www.medicalnewstoday.com. This potato is currently being sold primarily in Florida under the SunLite brand, www.sunfreshofflorida.com.

32. *"With protein spreads, the last couple of years have been just wild.":* S. Roesler, Minnesota Farm Guide, Posted: Friday, February 11, 2011 2:49 pm., accessed on February 26, 2012, http://minesotafarmguide.com/news/regional/experts-markets-paying-premiums-for-high-protein-wheat.

33. *"Obesity, diabetes mortality, and calorie consumption were associated with income inequality in developed countries":* K. Pickett, and others. "Wider income gaps, wider waistbands? An ecological study of obesity and income inequality," J Epidemiol Community Health 2005;59:670-674. Doi: 10.1136/jech.2004.028795.

34. *…most favorable Factor Condition on Planet Earth of 309,607,601 acres of rich Harvested Cropland (that's a USDA term)…:* USDA Economic Research Service, 2007 Census of Agriculture, accessed on January 17, 2012, http://www.ers.usda.gov/Search.aspx?searchTerm=census%20of%20agriculture.

35. *Here are Geoffrey Moore's two bell shaped curves.:* G. Moore, Crossing the Chasm. (New York: HarperBusiness, 1991), pp. 12-17.

36. *Percent of Adults Who Were Current Smokers*: CDC. National Center for Health Statistics. National Health Interview Survey 1965-2009. Analysis for years 1997-2009 by the American Lung Association, Research and Program Services using SPSS/PASW software.

37. *Percent of Adults Who Smoke by the Number of Cigarettes Smoked Daily*: CDC. National Center for Health Statistics. National Health Interview Survey. 1974-2009. Analysis for years 1997-2009 by the American Lung Association, Research and Program Services Division using SPSS and SUDAAN software.

38. *"...in the US, food manufacturers are permitted an error of plus or minus 20% when stating carbohydrate [and other Class II nutrients] content on product nutrition labels."*: R. Bernstein, *The Diabetes Diet* (New York: Little, Brown and Company, 2005), p. 31.

39. *...the "80/120 rule" can be found in FDA Regulation 21CFR101.9(g).*: FDA, "How Compliance Works—Title 21 of the Code of Federal Regulations (21 CFR 101.9(g))." Accessed in November 9, 2011, http://www.fda.gov/Food/Guidance-ComplianceRegulatoryInformation.

40. *"High-carbohydrate diet causes the pancreas to produce large amounts of insulin... leads to atherosclerosis and heart disease."*: Victoria Products, Accessed on October 31, 2011, http://www.victoriapacking.com/carb.html.

41. *...the obscene 17% administrative cost that is associated with our commercial health care system.*: masscare.org, accessed on March 5, 2012, http://mascare.org/health-care-costs/overhead-costs-of-health-care.

42. *...the administrative cost associated with Medicare is 5%.*: masscare.org, accessed on March 5, 2012, http://mascare.org/health-care-costs/overhead-costs-of-health-care.

43. *"Effective [diabetes, hypertension, smoking, and obesity] prevention could substantially improve the health of older Americans...with little or no additional lifetime medical spending."* D. Goldman and others, "The Benefits of Risk Factor Prevention in Americans Aged 51 Years and Older, American Journal of Public Health. 2009;99(1):2096, Posted 01/25/2010, accessed on January 15, 2012, http://www.medscape.com/viewarticle/71437.

CHAPTER 11: Let Freedom Ring –Again

1. *"In his latest effort to fight obesity in this era of Big Gulps… I don't want to pay more for health insurance so people can have these drinks!"*: S. Gross, Associated Press, Thursday, May 31, 2012 4:33 PM EDT.

2. *"Dr. Lustig treats sick, obese children, who he believes are primarily sick because of the amount of sugar they ingest… 'I think sugar belongs in this exact same wastebasket.'"*: "Is Sugar Toxic?" CBS News, March 30, 2012 1:00 PM. Accessed on March 31, 2012, http://www.cbsnews.com/2102-18560_162-57407128.html.

3. The spelling of Smith Thammasaroj varies.: The most frequent spelling is Thammasaroj. However, it also appears as Dharmasaroja and Dharmmasaroja.

4. *…he's the fellow who tried to prevent the deaths of 227,898…*: Wikipedia references a US Geological Survey, accessed on April 8, 2012, http://en.wikipedia.org/wiki/2004_Indian_Ocean_earthquake_and_tsunami.

5. *…innocent humans in 13 countries…*: Bangkok Post: Memory never fades, accessed on August 31, 2020, http://www.bangkokpost.com/business/economics/29678/memory-never-fades.

6. *"In September 1998,…media tended to disregard Smith's warnings, and even mocked him…saying there would surely be warnings and predictions if any natural disasters were about to occur."*: The Nation Opinion, Bangkok's Independent Newspaper, Published on March 23, 2005, accessed on August 31, 2010, http://nationalmultimedia.com/option/print.php?newsid= 113562.

7. *"Human safety was also sacrificed on the altar of tourist interests [big business] in Thailand in the last decade…One week after the tsunami the Prime Minister of Thailand, Thaksin Shinawatra, appointed [Smith] Thammasaroj as a minister in charge of the newly established national disaster warning office."*: Accessed on August 31, 2010, http://eapi.admu.edu.ph/content/people-faith-and-st-stephen%E2%80%99s-day-tsunami.

8. *"Now I can die in peace because what I warned has come true. Still, I feel sorry that I could not help save the lives of thousands of people."*: S. Wannabovorn in Bangkok, The Guardian, Wednesday 12 January 2005 00:02 GMT, accessed on August 31, 2010, http://www.guardian.co.uk/world/2005/jan/12/tsunami2004.thailand.

9. *Dr. Stephen D. Phinney, MD, PhD, is a physician-scientist who has spent 35 years studying diet, exercise, fatty acids, and inflammation and has published over 70 papers and several patents. He received his MD from Stanford University, his PhD in Nutritional Bio-Chemistry from MIT, and post-doctoral training at the University of Vermont and Harvard.*: J. Volek and S. Phinney. *The Art and Science of Low Carbohydrate Living* (2011), p. 279.

10. *If someone pulls this "cast doubt" routine, point out... "Increased consumption of refined carbohydrates and the epidemic of type 2 diabetes in the United States: an ecological assessment.".*: L. S. Gross and others. "Increased consumption of refined carbohydrates and the epidemic of type 2 diabetes in the United States: an ecological assessment," *Am J Clin Nutr* 2004; 79-774-9, accessed on February 16, 2012, http://www.ajcn.org.

11. *Then point out our federal government's NIH (National Institute of Health) website.*: National Institute of Diabetes and Digestive and Kidney Diseases (NIDDK), National Diabetes Statistics, 2011, Accessed July 15, 2012, http://diabetes.niddk.nih.gov/dm/pubs/statistics/index.aspx.

12. Ibid.

13. *By age 65, around two-thirds of all seniors have at least one chronic disease and see seven physicians. Twenty percent of those older than 65 have five or more chronic diseases, see 14 physicians – and average 40 doctor visits a year.*: A. D. Hoven, MD. Coping with baby boomers, and staggering statistics. AMA Leader Community, amednews.com. Posted September 20, 2010, accessed on July 10, 2012, http://www.ama-assn.org/amednews/2010/09/20/edca0920.htm.

14. *"Medicare costs to reduce Social Security increase. That didn't last long...millions of older Americans continue to struggle to make ends meet."*: S. Ohlemacher, Associated Press, October 19, 2011 6:12 PM EDT.

15. *"The next President and Congress may well determine the future of Medicare and Social Security. Don't let Washington make decisions about your future without hearing from you."*: Fred Griesbach, AARP Campaigns e-mail, sent April 10, 2012 05:00 AM.

16. *...we can leverage our 309,607,601...*: USDA Economic Research Service, 2007 Census of Agriculture, accessed on January 17, 2012, http://www.ers.usda.gov/Search.aspx?searchTerm=census%20of%20agriculture.

17. *The Low Cost of Corn in Food*: National Corn Growers Association, accessed on October 8, 2011. http://www.ncga.com/facts.

18. *"Transfer of technology could take time. There aren't enough officials to do this work. At the hobli [cluster of villages] level it is difficult even to get two officials. The university cannot take responsibility as we are already training, researching and doing technology transfer to a small extent."*: DNA/Shilpa C B / Tuesday, November 15, 2011 12:28 IST, accessed on February 25, 2012, http://www.dnaindia.com.

19. *...trade deficit with China - $295 billion in 2011.*: US Census. 2011: U.S. trade in goods with China, accessed on April 8, 2012, http://www.census.gov/foreign-trade/balance/c5700.html.

20. *...has eliminated or displaced 2.8 million U. S. jobs between 2001 and 2010.*: R. Scott, "Growing U.S. Trade Deficit with China Cost 2.8 million Jobs Between 2001 and 2010. Economic Policy Institute, September 20, 2011, Briefing Paper #323, www.epi.org.

21. *Here's the headline again, Export markets paying premiums for high protein wheat.*: S. Roesler, Minnesota Farm Guide, Posted: Friday, February 11, 2011 2:49 pm., accessed on February 26, 2012, http://minesotafarmguide.com/news/regional/experts-markets-paying-premiums-for-high-protein-wheat.

22. *...most farms are small (54.4% are less than 99 acres and 31% are less than 500 acres). The annual sales generated by these farms is miniscule (annually 59.8% generate <$10,000 and 18.3% generate <$50,000). And the vast majority of farms are owned by 1,906,335 individuals (86.5%) rather than big corporations.*: USDA Economic Research Service, 2007 Census of Agriculture, accessed on January 17, 2012, http://www.ers.usda.gov/Search.aspx?searchTerm=census%20of%20agriculture.

23. *...the pioneering innovation of a company called Generation UCAN.*: Accessed on July 24, 2012, http://generationucan.com/super.html.

24. *...the insulin response from consuming maltodextrin was nearly 8 times greater than that from consuming SuperStarch.*: Generation UCAN, accessed on May 20, 2012, http://generationucan.com/proof.html.

25. Ibid.

26. Ibid.

27. *An IRB is an appropriately constituted group that has been formally designated to review and monitor biomedical research involving human subjects.*: FDA, What is an Institutional Review Board(IRB)?, accessed on July 24, 2012, http://www.fda.gov/RegulatoryInformation/Guidances/ucm126420.htm.

28. *IRB's are responsible for critical oversight functions for research conducted on human subjects that are 'scientific', 'ethical', and 'regulatory'.*: Wikipedia, Institutional review board. Accessed on July 24, 2012, http://en.widipedia.org/wiki/Institutional_review_board.

29. *...UL was founded back in 1894...first test was conducted on March 24, 1984 on non-combustible insulation materials...*: Underwriter's Laboratory. Accessed on July 24, 2012, http://www.ul.com/global/eng/pages/corporate/aboutul.history.

30. *The UL Mark on a product means that UL has tested and evaluated representative samples of that product and determined that they meet UL requirements.*: Underwriter's Laboratory. Accessed on July 24, 2012, http://www.ul.com/global/eng/pages/corporate/aboutul/ulmarks.

31. *Today, there are dozens of UL marks made for Asia, Europe, Latin America, and North America.*: Underwriter's Laboratory. Accessed on July 24, 2012, http://www.ul.com/global/eng/pages/corporate/aboutul/ulmarks/mark.

32. *In 2011, 22.4 billion UL Marks appeared on products made by 67,798 manufacturers around the globe.*: Underwriter's Laboratory. Accessed on July 24, 2012, http://ul.com/global/eng/pages/corporate/aboutul.

33. *...according to diabetes expert Richard K. Bernstein, MD, some foods that say they have few or zero carbs actually cause a significant insulin response in humans.*: R. Bernstein. *Dr. Bernstein's Diabetes Solution* (New York: Little, Brown and Company, 2011), pp. 150-152.

34. *Mitochondria are the little sausage-shaped organelles inside the cells that convert the energy stored in food to ATP, the energy currency of the body.*: M.R. Eades, MD. Accessed on July 24, 2012, http://www.proteinpower.com/drmike/weight-loss/mitochondria-rejuvenating-diet-the-nutritional-experts-bash.

35. *"To facilitate fat utilization, muscle triglycerides in trained individuals [athletes] are localized near mitochondria...decreased number and size of mitochondria and overall reduced oxidative capacity in the untrained obese person."*: J. Volek and S. Phinney. *The Art and Science of Low Carbohydrate Living* (2011), p. 182.

36. *Then there's Dr. Terry Wahls MD, a physician who was struck down by a relent-lessly progressive neurodegenerative disorder. It's called MS or Multiple Sclerosis... I strongly encourage you to watch her 17 minute YouTube video.*: Accessed on August 6, 2012, http://www.youtube.com/watch?v=KLjgBLwH3Wc.

37. *"Studies from all over the world have consistently shown that, when used as the first treatment, about 60% of children will have at least a 50% reduction in their seizures within 6 months....which can suppress seizures."*: J. Volek and S. Phinney. *The Art and Science of Low Carbohydrate Living* (2011), pp. 251-252.

38. *"In my opinion, The Art and Science of Low Carbohydrate Living [self-published] is simply the best how-to book on low-carb dieting...the editor would force the authors to change it."*: M. R. Eades, MD. Accessed on August 6, 2012, http://www.protein-power.com/drmike/saturated-fat/the-best-low-carb-book-in-print.

39. *...features Dr. Robert Lustig, MD, the pediatrician who says that "sugar not only leads to obesity, but to Type 2 diabetes, hypertension and heart disease itself."*: "Is Sugar Toxic?" CBS News, March 30, 2012 1:00 PM. Accessed on March 31, 2012, http://www.cbsnews.com/2102-18560_162-57407128.html.

40. *According to their website, "Smoker Friendly® is completely dedicated to the sale and promotion of cigarettes, cigars, all other tobacco products and related smoker's accessories in our stores through our friendly and knowledgeable store opera-tors."*: Accessed on March 20, 2012, http://www.smokerfriendly.com/customer.cfm?pageName=About.

41. *I still can't believe the old McDonalds 22 oz. Chocolate McCafe Shake used to con-tain 147 grams of carbs!*: McDonald's USA NutritionFacts for Popular Menu Items, PDF, saved on March 30, 2012.

42. *"The Americans were underdogs, but they were competitive. [Coach] Brooks suggest-ed that a bronze medal was within reach."*: J. Fitzpatrick, Miracle on Ice: American Hockey's Defining Moment, About.com, accessed on June 26, 2012, http://proice-hockey.about.com/cs/history/a/miracle_on_ice.htm.

INDEX

www.ingramcontent.com/pod-product-compliance
Lightning Source LLC
Chambersburg PA
CBHW081145270326
41930CB00014B/3043